Now regarded as a leading authority in her field, Christina Maslach was one of the first psychologists to explore the burnout phenomenon. She holds a Ph.D. in social psychology from Stanford University and is an associate professor at the University of California-Berkeley. In addition to teaching, she has done extensive research on the subject of burnout and has written several books and many articles in such publications as *Psychology Today*.

Philip G. Zimbardo, author of the prologue, is a professor of psychology at Stanford University and has written many books, including the best-seller *Shyness* and *Psychology and Life*.

Now regarded as a leading authority in her field, Christina Maslach was one of the first psychologists to explore the burnout phenomenon. She holds a Ph.D. in social psychology from Stanford University and is an associate professor at the University of California, Berkeley. In addition to teaching, she has done extensive research on the subject of burnout and has written several books and many articles in such publications as *Psychology Today*.

Philip G. Zimbardo, author of the prologue, is a professor of psychology at Stanford University and has written many books, including the best-seller *Shyness* and *Psychology and Life*.

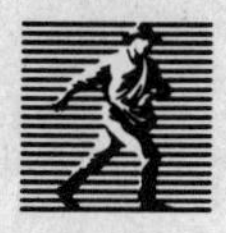

PRENTICE HALL PRESS
New York London Toronto Sydney Tokyo

CHRISTINA MASLACH
prologue by Philip G. Zimbardo

BURNOUT
THE COST OF CARING

To my parents,
George J. Maslach and Doris C. Maslach,
whose love and caring
have meant so much to me

Published in 1986 by Prentice Hall Press
A Division of Simon & Schuster, Inc.
Gulf + Western Building
One Gulf + Western Plaza
New York, NY 10023

Originally published by Prentice-Hall, Inc.
Cover design by Jeannette Jacobs
Cover illustration by Uri Salzman

Library of Congress Cataloging-in-Publication Data

Maslach, Christina.
Burnout, the cost of caring.

Bibliography: p.
Includes index
1. Burn out (Psychology) I. Title. [DNLM: 1. Stress, Psychological. 2. Job satisfaction. WM 172 M397b]
BF481.M384 1982 158.7 82-9057
AACR2
ISBN 0-13-091231-X (pbk.)

Manufactured in the United States of America

17 16 15 14 13 12 11 10 9

CONTENTS

ACKNOWLEDGMENTS

Many people have played important roles in this analysis of burnout. Foremost among them is Susan E. Jackson, who has collaborated with me on numerous research studies and on the development of the Maslach Burnout Inventory. She is a superb researcher, a wonderful colleague, and a good friend—and I am deeply grateful for all that she has done. I also want to give a special thanks to the people who helped me begin this research: Kathy Kelly Moore, who first "discovered" burnout with me and who has continued to provide thoughtful comments; Ayala Pines, who was a valued collaborator on the first survey studies of burnout; Maxine Gann, whose clinical expertise has extended my own thinking about this problem; and Steve Heckman, whose experience and sensitivity to various issues in burnout have added much to my understanding of this syndrome. I am indebted to several research assistants whose work was especially helpful: Herschel Kwinter, Elizabeth Lopez, Jennifer Chatman, Cheryl Arnott, Amy Honigman, and Christina Zoppel. Many other students at the University of California at Berkeley participated in various phases of the research program, from planning discussions and library research to the collection and coding of data, and I wish to thank all of them for their time and efforts. I also appreciate the research funding provided by several Biomedical Sciences Support Grants.

I owe a special debt of gratitude to the many individuals who shared their experiences with me and gave me permission to quote them in this book. Their eloquent statements truly enrich and give life to the abstract ideas and research findings that I discuss here. I also want to thank Cheryl Wade for her excellent work on the annotated bibliography.

Finally, this book would not have come into being without a very special person—my husband and colleague, Phil Zimbardo. From the beginning, he has been strong in his encouragement and constructive in his criticisms and has made many important contributions to my writing. His warmth, good humor, patience, and understanding have kept me going even when the going got tough. The love and support that he and our daughters, Zara and Tanya, have given me throughout this period have kept my own fire burning brightly, and for that I am truly grateful.

PROLOGUE by Philip G. Zimbardo

THREE STORIES: RONNIE, SNUFFY, AND CHRIS

My cousin, Ronnie Petrillo, is a cop, a good cop, honored for bravery, liked by his buddies, still an idealist about preserving law and order and making his beat a safer place for people to live.[1]

My friend Snuffy Thompson, is a robber, a bad robber, who gets arrested a lot, goes to prison some of the time, cons gullible souls into paying big money for worthless jewelry or someone else's Cadillac–and back to the slammer for a while.

As different as the two of them are, I think you'd like them both if they'd let you get on the good side of their tough hides. Ronnie and Snuffy each play cameo roles in the tragic drama entitled "Burnout." The cop is but one of the many kinds of other actors you will soon meet, whose life's work entails providing a service to people in need. They are professional providers, the caregivers in our drama—health care, educational care, welfare care, legal care, and whatever other kind of care one can make a career out of giving. Their stage directions call for "close contact" with the receivers of their services. Although cautioned about getting "too close" or making "too much contact," these actors sometimes fail to maintain a sufficiently detached perspective. When this happens the role gets to them, and they no longer can tell where the role ends and the self begins, or is it the self ends and the role takes over?

Snuffy is on the receiving end. He "gets done to" by these providers of people services. Cops track him down and arrest him, lawyers defend him, guards try to control him, prison counselors attempt to straighten him out, parole agents keep tabs on his activities, welfare personnel help him survive until the next time, and so on and so forth. But Snuffy is just one of a cast of millions who are the recipients of care from the ever-growing human services industry in our country. Care that used to come informally from individuals in our tribe, our family, our neighborhood, from the elders, now is packaged more formally by institutions with trained staffs of personnel who specialize in giving particular kinds of care to particular kinds of recipients, or cynically, the "care-takers."

Ronnie and Snuffy have interesting stories to tell about how "the system" can work against, rather than for, them. But before we check out their stories, I should mention that the author of the drama that is about to unfold in this book, Christina Maslach, also has a little side story that needs telling. She won't do it herself because of her sense of professional modesty, so I will have to because of my personal pride. It's the kind of story that reveals a hidden dimension of a person whom we thought we really knew until something totally unexpected happened and the person improvised on the spot—sometimes for better, as in this case, or for worse, as in too many other instances. Since Ronnie and Snuffy are already stage center, let's put Christina's story aside for the moment.

Ronnie

I've known Ronnie since he was a little kid, an easy-going, fun-loving kid. Full of smarts, but short on the discipline "to study hard to get into college like your cousin Philip." He had a variety of jobs that were fillers until he found what he really wanted to do with his life. When he finally became a police officer, at last he found the right career for his talents and interests. He was doing something for his community, not just working at a meaningless job selling some product only for the commission it brought.

"I help people who are weak, frightened, and in trouble. Thugs don't harass the shopkeepers in my area, junkies think twice before dealing around the school. Old ladies don't have to be in constant fear of their Social Security checks being ripped off. I'm only sorry that violence is so much a part of the job. We are the lightning rods that deflect the bullets and abuse from some target out there in the community onto us. And then we may have to kick ass to keep some hood from killing one of us or one of you."

The emergency call blasts in on his car radio. "'Signal 21' [burglary in progress], culprit 'signal zone' [believed armed], still on premises. All units in area proceed to scene immediately; Unit 57 is closest and will be contact unit to enter premises. Unit 23 backup in rear yard, Unit 14 cover roof. Over and out."

Adrenaline flows in tune with wailing siren. "I'll go in, you hit it last time, cover for me, stay in real close." Heartbeat in ears almost drums out all other sounds. "This is the police. Come out with your arms above your head and you will not be harmed." Silence. Pulse racing. Door kicked in. No resistance. No suspect. Room by room the apartment is searched for the dangerous suspect who could be hiding in a closet or behind a shower curtain–with a nervous finger on a fast trigger.

"No one's here, premises empty." "Relief! False alarm, or did the bad guy make a quick escape? But what do I do with all this pumped up adrenaline? How do I push that pulse down to its old resting place?"

Ronnie overreacts a little in subduing a known drug dealer caught red-handed. He snarls back, "I'm gonna get you, you fag mother fucker, soon as I'm out!"

"That's the second citizen complaint against you this week, Petrillo. I've had some community leaders in here who are distressed by the way you handled a forcible arrest in their neighborhood. Apparently, you lost control of the situation. I can't tolerate that kind of . . ."

"But Chief, a crowd of 200 people threatened us, they were going to take away our suspect, who was one of three bad guys who jumped another cop. We were lucky to escape from there alive.

"OK, sure, Chief, next time we'll handle it differently. But I gotta tell you, you've been off the streets too long, you don't have any idea what we are up against out there. It would be nice to know that we had a little support from somewhere, but we don't seem to have any, not from the DA's office, or the judges, or top brass. We're alone out there and it's cold."

Sure, it's past shift time, but there are still a mass of forms to be completed before heading home. Five A.M., the sun is coming up as Ronnie leaves the station house. "Can I buy you a cup of coffee, Copper? Told you it was a waste of time. I'm bailed out already before you even got to bed! And while you're sleeping, I'll make more money than you pick up in a month doing your Boy Scout errands." Frustration, anger. Some of it turned out, some turned in.

"He's getting like a real Gestapo when he puts that uniform on," my mother told me. "He's always yelling at the kids, ordering everybody around, no patience at all, can't stand any noise." "We're all on pins and needles when he's home," his wife reports. "Ronnie doesn't eat good like he used to, it's those night shifts and junk food. He's coming in to sleep when we're all getting ready to start the day. But he hasn't been sleeping so good lately either, and that makes him even more irritable and more exhausted when he's got to work overtime because somebody else calls in sick. And how can we have any social life with these hours?"

Ronnie sighs, "The headaches I handle with aspirin, Gelusil for the stomach aches, and a drink for the nerves. It seemed to be working until last Sunday when I noticed my speech slurring and my hand getting numb, then my arm and the right side of my face. I had a stroke. Imagine me with a stroke. I'm not even forty years old, and I got a stroke. Maybe it's the stress of the job, who knows, but what's new? It's part of my job. Fortunately, the stroke went away with a little rest and medication in the hospital. Doctor said I should take it easy. 'I'll try, doc, but I can't promise. I mean, to be a cop is to be a stress officer. It's what the job is all about. If I can't cope out there, I might as well be a night watchman in a cemetery.' I guess I've just got to get tougher so the job doesn't get to me the way it does. But *how* to do that is another matter."

Snuffy

Snuffy is not only the kind of person who makes Ronnie's job a source of so much stress, he is the "client" who contributes his fair share to increasing the emotional exhaustion in a host of other caregivers. He certainly exhausts my emotional reserves at times, gives me a case of *agita* (Sicilian for a state of aggravated irritability, the best cure for which is to bite one's lips, count to *dieci*, and exit from the situation *presto*). Snuffy's endless litany of problems, complaints, imagined injustices, his broken promises, missed appointments, unpredictable outbursts tax not only my patience, but almost everything else in and around me. There are times, I am ashamed to admit, that I wish he would just go away, vanish, or be banished to a desert island without access to the phone that he calls me on at midnight to ask for advice on how to deal with the welfare worker who won't process his request for supplementary aid. He threatened to do her in if she didn't wise up. You see he really needs the money to pay his lawyer who got him off a drunk driving charge ("How can a couple of shots get you drunk? I mean to tell you, those cops are out to get me because I don't take no shit from them, they can't come on my turf pushing us around. If I'm gonna do time again, I'm taking a few of them with me").

The welfare agent pressed the panic button, security subdued Snuffy, who was irate that he should be treated like a common criminal. "Lady, your time will come, don't ever forget my face because next time you see it, it will be too late." She didn't know he was more puff than tough stuff. The parole officer managed to get Snuffy released with the promise of psychiatric counseling. But the clinic psychiatrist did not have enough street savvy to rap on a par with Snuffy's fast talk, so Snuffy dismissed him as another of the incompetents "full of book learning, but without any common sense." "I told him he was a dunce when it came to really understanding people. I gave him a D grade; come back when you're ready to get down in human terms." Parole revoked, some county jail time. Guards are made to pay for the fact that nobody wants to give Snuffy a break, start him out with a decent stake, let him run a small business, give him a franchise, or whatever. And it's their fault too that "rich kids are born with a silver spoon in their mouths and the children of the poor get lead poisoning from the peeling paint off the rotten walls of their rat-infested tenements that are there to make fat-cat landlords fatter and make jobs for those 'home-relief workers.' That's what they used to be called in the old days in New York, now they are social welfare pukes."

And that's just a week in the life of Snuffy Thompson. As his world turns so do the stomachs of the half dozen or more professional service providers he uses and abuses. They are not part of his solution, according to him, and he is definitely part of their problem, according to them.

People needing people. People unable to make it on their own. People wanting to help others to cope, to survive, to adapt, to adjust, to make it. It is a reaching out and a making contact. It is the human connection. It brings a sense of fulfillment to the givers, to the sharers of their talents and energies. It brings relief, help, direction, new beginnings to those who take that hand being offered. When it works, this human drama is a joy to behold. When it doesn't work, it can be comic, but all too often it is tragic. The givers suffer, and those in need are not helped as they should be. The human connection is not renewed with gentle, firm human contact. It is broken or frozen with callous disregard and cynical disappointment: "So that's what those people are really like—they're animals, that's what they are, animals."

Christina Maslach deftly leads us through the various acts in which this tragic drama of the work place develops. We are shown how the principal actors and actresses are affected by the stresses of the setting in which they work, what each contributes to the problem, and how each spreads its insidious malaise to others. But just when the stage appears strewn with the burnt offerings of once overzealous performers, our author redirects the action to suggest not only ways to rekindle the flame of the caregivers, but, even more, to discover how to prevent it from beginning to flicker. The end, however, awaits writing, since the author rightly notes that recommendations need to be translated into scripts for action, actions made into policy, policy outcomes evaluated, and evaluations appraised to guide further interventions.

The optimist in me holds out for an idyllic final scene, which when eventually written will be that "the worker enjoyed the work, those helped enjoyed the helpers and were enjoyed in return as problems found their rightful solutions and solutions ended unfair problems. And burnout disappeared from the land as people rediscovered the joy in giving and receiving the help, care, and concern that we all need at times in our journey through life."

You are now close to meeting the author who you will find most knowledgeable about the actors and the contexts in which they perform. She has researched her subject well and makes her knowledge readily accessible by using language that is both common and precise. Thus laypeople, professional caregivers, and social scientists (among others in her audience) will all be able to take away much from this unpretentious scholarly analysis that is informed by the obvious personal involvement of a researcher who seeks to understand and a gentle, caring person who would use that understanding to improve the lives of others.

Chris

Finally, Chris's story. Some years ago I was a prison superintendent. I ran the Stanford County Prison, an experimental prison created by psychologists to study the dynamics of the prisoner-guard relationship. Our mock prison was populated with "good guards" and "good prisoners"; we knew that was so because we rigged it that way. Only normal, healthy, law-abiding volunteers were selected to role play being jailers or inmates. A flip of the coin randomly segregated the lot into opposing sides, so that there was no basis in reality for any person to be a prisoner or a guard. But like a Pirandello play, the illusion we created soon merged with reality. Our mock prison became all too real. Guards who were generally passive and pacifist became sadistic and brutal. Prisoners chosen for their "normalcy" on a variety of personality tests were behaving pathologically in a variety of ways. The mere fact of a prisoner's existence in the prison justified degradation by the guards. Prisoners deserved what they got because they were "troublemakers" and "dangerous." The worst abuses to the inmates occurred when the prison officials were asleep or otherwise occupied, when a guard was alone with a prisoner—when the "experiment" was suspended and personal motives took over. Mind you, everyone knew this had started out as an experiment, but that memory grew less vivid as each day passed.

The inmates were awakened several times a night, allegedly to be counted, but really so the night shift guards could have something to do to keep from being bored. By the time parents and friends visited, most inmates looked awful and felt terrible. A priest visited and watched as a prisoner broke down sobbing hysterically. A public defender interviewed prisoners who complained about the conditions of their incarceration. Secretaries, psychologists, people from TV and news media, janitors, and assorted others looked in from time to time to see this evil place gradually overwhelm those good people acting out their assigned roles.

I thought of myself as a "liberal administrator"; indeed, some guards complained that I was too soft with the prisoners. By the fifth night all of us were caught up in the escalation of power to the powerful, the suffering of the powerless, and the need to control people (rather than scientific variables). In this hothouse atmosphere, I had not realized the transformation that was taking place in me—me the dispassionate researcher, the always eager-to-please teacher, the liberal prison superintendent. I had changed, I was now the zoo keeper, the menagerie manager, and these were my trained, tamed animals.

Christina brought that realization crashing down on me with a tear. It was Thursday night and she came to the prison to assist us with interviewing the prisoners. While she was preparing the tape recorder and interview materials, I called her attention to the line of blindfolded prisoners, shuffling along to the toilet under the guard's orders. She averted her eyes, and when I asked had she seen the *prisoners* (our "circus"), she tearfully replied, "It's awful what you are doing to those boys." Hers was the first voice in nearly a week to break through the reality of "our prison" to remind us that they were boys, not prisoners, that they had not done anything to justify what we were doing to them, and that the experiment was out of control. Not a single person of the more than thirty observers who came to peep in (through the observation window) at our study, nor any of the dozen parents and friends of the prisoners who came on two visiting nights, had questioned the basic assumptions of our prison. Christina's tears cut through the "groupthink" consensus that had isolated us from external normative standards and from our own moral and human values. Hers was the gentle voice that reminded me of my humanity, of the distance I had traveled blindly to become what this place and that role dictated. Her courage to challenge the entire irrational system was sufficient to force me to end it the next day, a week before the projected termination day. We had traveled too far, the momentum of the place had prevailed over our sense and sensibility.

Christina Maslach's courage was all the greater considering that she also had to break through the constraints of her role as mere graduate student to challenge not only the formidable prison superintendent, but a man who was her professor and thesis supervisor as well.

There was only one obvious course of action open for me in responding to this affront to my authority—I married her. And now there is only one obvious course of action open to you, dear reader: to get acquainted with this remarkable woman through her perceptive analysis of the phenomenon of burn-out. Curtain!

1

THE BURNOUT SYNDROME

When I try to describe my experience to someone else, I use the analogy of a teapot. Just like a teapot, I was on the fire, with water boiling—working hard to handle problems and do good. But after several years, the water had boiled away, and yet I was still on the fire—a burned-out teapot in danger of cracking.

Carol B., social worker

A teacher can be compared to a battery. At the beginning of the school year, all the students are plugged in and drawing learning current. At the end of the school year, the battery is worn down and must be recharged. And each time the battery is recharged it is more difficult to get it to hold its charge, and eventually it must be replaced. That is when complete burnout has taken place.

Jim Y., teacher

When you have to care for so many people, you begin to suffer from an emotional overload—it's just too much. I'm like a wire that has too much electricity flowing through it—I've burned out and emotionally disconnected from others."

Jane J., nurse

Burnout. The word evokes images of a final flickering flame, of a charred and empty shell, of dying embers and cold, gray ashes. And, indeed, these images aptly express what these three people, Carol, Jim, and Jane, are now experiencing. All of them were once fired up about their involvement with other people—excited, full of energy, dedicated, willing to give tremendously of themselves for others. And they *did* give . . . and give, and give until finally there was nothing left to give anymore. The teapot was empty, the battery was drained, the circuit was overloaded—they had burned out.

Burnout is a syndrome of emotional exhaustion, depersonalization, and reduced personal accomplishment that can occur among individuals who do "people work" of some kind. It is a response to the chronic emotional strain of dealing extensively with other human beings, particularly when they are troubled or having problems. Thus, it can be considered one type of job stress. Although it has some of the same deleterious effects as other stress responses, what is unique about burnout is that the stress arises from the *social* interaction between helper and recipient.

A pattern of emotional overload and subsequent emotional exhaustion is at the heart of the burnout syndrome. A person gets overly involved emotionally, overextends him- or herself, and feels overwhelmed by the emotional demands imposed by other people. The response to this situation (and thus one aspect of burnout) is *emotional exhaustion.* People feel drained and used up. They lack enough energy to face another day. Their emotional resources are depleted, and there is no source of replenishment. As Betty G. put it, "Everyday I was knocking myself out at school—for the kids primarily, but also to prove to others (and myself) that I was a good teacher. I would really be emotionally drained, but all I had to come home to was the cat." Her motto might have been, "I gave at the office—who will give me something back?"

Once emotional exhaustion sets in, people feel they are no longer able to give of themselves to others. "It's not that I don't want to help, but that I can't—I seem to have a 'compassion fatigue.' I just can't motivate myself to climb one more mountain." One way people try to get out from under their emotional burden is by cutting back on their involvement with others. They want to reduce their contact with people to the bare minimum required to get the job done. Consequently, they transform themselves into petty bureaucrats whose dealings with people go strictly by the book. They "pigeonhole" people into various categories and then respond to the category rather than to the individual. By applying a formula, rather than a unique response, they avoid having to get to know the other person and becoming emotionally involved.

This petty bureaucrat routine is one of the many ways people detach themselves psychologically from any meaningful involvement with others. This detachment puts some emotional distance between oneself and the people whose needs and demands are overwhelming. When this emotional buffer is combined with a genuine caring for others, it evolves into an effective way of handling the emotional strain of such people work. The professional ideal of "detached concern" among medical practitioners represents this blend of closeness and distance.[1] Many physicians believe it is a prerequisite for effective patient care. But, much like oil and water, detachment and concern do not mix easily. Rather than striking and sustaining a balance between them, many people feel pulled toward one or the other of these apparently antithetical poles. All too often, the professional's commitment to helping is so overwhelming that the retreat into a detached stance toward others is actually an attempt at emotional self-protection—patients get care or treatment without any personal caring.

The armor of detachment may indeed shield the individual from the strain of close involvement with others, but it can also be so thick that no feeling gets through. With increasing detachment comes an attitude of cold indifference to others' needs and a callous disregard for their feelings. As one New York cop told me:

> You change when you become a cop—you become tough and hard and cynical. You have to condition yourself to be that way in order to survive this job. And sometimes, without realizing it, you act that way all the time, even with your wife and kids. But it's something you have to do, because if you start getting emotionally involved with what happens at work, you'll wind up in Bellevue [psychiatric hospital].

The development of this detached, callous, and even dehumanized response signals a second aspect of the burnout syndrome—*depersonalization.* It is as though the individual is viewing other people through rust-colored glasses—developing a poor opinion of them, expecting the worst from them, and even actively disliking them. According to one social worker, "I began to despise everyone and could not conceal my contempt," while another reports, "I find myself caring less and possessing an extremely negative attitude. I just don't give a damn anymore." This increasingly negative reaction to people manifests itself in various ways. The provider may derogate other people and put them down, refuse to be civil and courteous to them, ignore their pleas and demands, or fail to provide the appropriate help, care, or service. Listen to Michelle B.'s experience:

> I'm a United States consul and am not alone among consular officers in experiencing burnout. We interview nonimmigrant visa applicants to determine whether they are eligible for visas and whether they are really nonimmigrants or intend to remain illegally in the United States. The poor will try any form of fraud or misrepresentation to get a visitor or student visa if they cannot qualify under the law. Weeding out the intending immigrants wouldn't be such a bad job, if it were not for the fact that we have about three minutes per interview, with hundreds more applicants clamoring for their turn. It's easy to dehumanize the applicants. We speak of cattle chutes to control the crowds. We lose our temper and yell at the refused applicants who won't give up and go away. We refuse visas because the

applicants have greasy hair or wide lapels. We refuse so many that we don't bother to tell applicants who could qualify for a waiver of ineligibility that there is such a thing. We begin to despise the poor, if not all nationals of the country we work in.

When the individual becomes soured by the press of humanity, he or she wishes, at times, that other people would "get out of my life and just leave me alone." In some cases, this wish is acted on, and the other people are literally shut out. As an example, it is not uncommon in residential colleges for faculty initially to encourage their students to come to their apartment in the dorm at any hour. However, when one student's problems are replayed over and over by many others, students themselves become the problem for the faculty member. Long before the school year ends, faculty begin to resent the students from whom there seems to be no escape. You can see why a student would then become thoroughly confused by a display of disdain from a teacher who had once been so friendly and helpful. Ironically, these hostile and negative feelings are often directed at the people one cares about most of all. As one harried young mother of three children put it: "There are days when I've had it up to here with talking to little people who are always whining and wanting something. And I'll be angry all the time, wishing they would just disappear."

Feeling negatively about others can progress until it encompasses being down on oneself. Caregivers feel distress or guilt about the way they have thought about or mistreated others. They sense they are turning into the very type of person—cold and uncaring—that nobody, especially them, likes very much. At this point, a third aspect of burnout appears—a feeling of *reduced personal accomplishment.* Providers have a gnawing sense of inadequacy about their ability to relate to recipients, and this may result in a self-imposed verdict of "failure." "It's painful to say it, but maybe I'm just not cut out for this kind of work," said one attorney in legal services. "I thought of myself as a sensitive and caring person, but often I'm *not* sensitive and caring when I'm with clients—so maybe I'm really deluding myself about the real me." With the crumbling of self-esteem, depression may set in, and some will seek counseling or therapy for what they believe are their personal problems. Others will change their jobs, often to abandon any kind of work that brings them into stressful contact with people.

A vivid example of a full-blown bout with burnout is Stan's experience:

I am a psychologist, going on my third year of employment as a therapist in a community mental health center. I have seen myself change from an avid, eager, open-minded, caring person to an extremely cynical, not-giving-a-damn individual in just two and a half years. I'm only twenty-six, and I've already developed an ulcer from doing continuous work in crisis intervention. I've gone through drinking to relax enough to go to sleep, tranquilizers, stretching my sick leave to its ultimate limit, and so on. At this point, to get through the year, I've chosen to flip into the attitude of going to the mental health center as if I were working at GM, Delco, or Frigidaire factories–that's what it has become here, a mental health *factory!* I am slowly, painfully beginning to realize that I need time away from constantly dealing with other people's sorrows, and that in order to head off the deadness that is beginning to happen inside of me, I must get away, apply for a month or so leave of absence, maybe more–when I start shaking just upon entering the office, then I know *that's it.* It hurts to feel like a failure as a therapist in terms of not being able to handle the pressure, but it's better that I do something about it now, rather than commit suicide later after letting it build up much longer.

"AT RISK" FOR BURNOUT

In listening to Stan, our first reaction is to ask, "Why did it happen?" Here is an intelligent and sensitive young man who was initially dedicated to a career of helping people, who had received some special training for such work, and who had started his job with a great deal of enthusiasm. He was, perhaps, the ideal person for this line of work–just the sort of caring and committed therapist that you and I would want to turn to in times of trouble. So why did he burn out?

Although he was not aware of it at the time, Stan's work situation made him clearly "at risk" for burnout. It required him to deal with many other people over an extended period of time. Hour after hour, day after day, he was supposed to help people with their "sorrows" and problems. And in doing so he was expected always to be concerned, warm, and caring. The emotional strain of such extensive caring was something he had underestimated or perhaps had not even recognized. He began to get too involved in his clients' woes and to feel overwhelmed by them. Added to this was a lack of rapport and support among his co-workers and administrators, an excess of paperwork and the frustrations of red tape. Thus, Stan was in a situation of escalating emotional overload–too much was being asked of him and too little was being returned to him. The inner flame of concern and caring that he had brought to his job was slowly being snuffed out.

Many other life situations, both at work and at home, share the same elements that Stan faced–and we will see that burnout is the typical consequence. Consider a teacher who must educate a class of thirty students; deal with all of their personal and social needs on a daily basis; discipline, influence, shape, manage, and direct their behavior over long hours–and then face possible friction and hostility from parents, the uncertainty of layoffs from administrators, and the ever-present threat of budget cutbacks from the community. Such a teacher is at risk for burnout. A mother who must care for several young children at home, without help or support from others, with no opportunity for a work break, is at risk for burnout. A minister who must be a source of refuge and support for anyone seeking help at any time, and who has no one to turn to when personal problems arise, is at risk for burnout. A police officer who deals continuously with the seamy side of life, with lawbreakers and victims of crime, with violence and potential danger lurking in every encounter with a stranger, is at risk for burnout. A doctor who wades in an unending stream of patients who are sick, upset, angry, and frightened by their illness or its implications, is also at risk for burnout. These are but a few of the many whose life's work makes them vulnerable to the emotional exhaustion, depersonalization, and reduced personal accomplishment that together form the burnout syndrome.

A PERSONAL ANALYSIS

This book represents my own ideas and insights about burnout. It is a personal analysis based on ten years of research and reflection. In collaboration with my colleagues at the University of California at Berkeley, I have collected information from thousands of people across the United States, by questionnaires, interviews, personal letters, or on-site observations. These individuals have come from a wide range of people-work occupations; they include social workers, teachers, police officers, nurses, physicians, psychotherapists, counselors, psychiatrists, ministers, child-care workers, mental health workers, prison personnel, legal services attorneys, psychiatric nurses, probation officers, and agency administrators. Although they perform different jobs, they all have in common extensive contact with other people in situations that are often emotionally charged.

At the time I began to study burnout, in the early 1970s, almost nothing was known about it. Few words had been written about the topic, and research on it was nonexistent. With so little to go on, I had no preconceived notions about burnout, nor did I have a particular theory that I wanted to prove. Instead, I had to start from scratch and take a very exploratory approach, in which I asked lots of questions and watched what people were doing. As I thought about all these bits and pieces of information, I saw a meaningful pattern emerging. I tried out my initial ideas at a national convention in 1973.[2] I then developed a working concept of the burnout process, which I described in *Human Behavior* magazine in 1976.[3] The public response to this article was overwhelming. Thousands of letters and telephone calls poured in from all parts of the United States and Canada. People wanted more information about burnout, some asked for help with their specific difficulties, and some expressed relief that at last this taboo topic had been made public. The article was reprinted or abstracted in many newspapers, magazines, and books; circulated widely in dozens of professional newsletters; assigned as required reading for various training and in-service programs; and distributed as a special handout at workshops and conventions. Clearly, burnout was a major concern for many people; it was as if a raw nerve had been touched.

As I continued to study burnout, my research began to involve more systematic tests of these initial ideas. The first two studies were done in collaboration with Ayala Pines, and investigated burnout among day-care workers[4] and mental health staff.[5] Subsequent studies were done in collaboration with Susan E. Jackson, and focused on legal services attorneys,[6] police officers,[7] physicians and nurses,[8] and public contact employees in the Social Security Administration.[9] To assess people's experience of burnout, Susan E. Jackson and I developed a standardized scale measure, the Maslach Burnout Inventory (MBI).[10] The MBI measures the three aspects of the burnout syndrome–emotional exhaustion, depersonalization, and reduced personal accomplishment–and is now the most widely used index of burnout in both research studies and organizational programs. The following outline gives sample items for each of these three components and indicates how frequently these feelings occur when burnout is high and when it is low.

THE MASLACH BURNOUT INVENTORY (MBI)[11]

Emotional Exhaustion subscale

- Sample items:
  - I feel emotionally drained from my work.
  - Working with people all day is really a strain for me.
- Frequency patterns:
  - High burnout–several times a month or more
  - Low burnout–several times a year or less

Depersonalization subscale

- Sample items:
  - I've become more callous toward people since I took this job.
  - I worry that this job is hardening me emotionally.
- Frequency patterns:
  - High burnout–once a month or more
  - Low burnout–once or twice a year, or less

Personal Accomplishment subscale (reverse scoring)

- Sample items:
  - In my work, I deal with emotional problems very calmly.
  - I feel I'm positively influencing other people's lives through my work.
- Frequency patterns:
  - High burnout–less than once a week
  - Low burnout–several times a week or daily

Each of my research projects has tried to fill in a piece of the burnout puzzle. As new information has come in, my ideas about burnout have developed and changed,[12] until they have culminated in the thesis in this book.

What I will be presenting here is a personal perspective based on a synthesis of all my research. I will not be giving a detailed discussion of specific research results; readers interested in reviewing the original data are referred to the articles listed in the annotated bibliography. Instead, I will be painting a more global picture of burnout as I have come to understand it, laying out major themes and issues. Central to my analysis is the distinction between *who* and *what*—that is, between individual people and the surrounding situation.

THE WHO VERSUS WHAT OF BURNOUT

When burnout begins to occur, whether in ourselves or in others, we tend to see *people* causing it. We blame either the provider or the recipient of care (or perhaps both) for spoiling the idealistic relationship between concerned giver and appreciative beneficiary of that gift. Something about *them* as people, some personal flaw, must be the source of their soured altruism—or so we think. "He's a cold fish." "She hasn't got a brain in her head." "I guess I'm just a real SOB." "You have to be crazy to be a psychiatrist." "What can you expect from cops? They're all sadists to begin with." These are the sorts of conclusions we come up with when trying to figure out who is causing the problem. But note that I've phrased the question in terms of *who.* Who is to blame for burnout? Who is responsible? Who caused this to happen? Whenever we ask a "who" question, what we get back will be a "who" answer. In other words, we will always conclude that it is a person or group of people who are the problem. Who? Me! Who? Them!

But suppose I pose the question differently: *What* is causing burnout? Phrased in these terms, the question points us in other directions that encourage us to substitute an analytical microscope for our people-watching binoculars. Rather than looking just at "defective" people, we focus our attention on the *situation* in which they find themselves. What sorts of tasks are they expected to do and why; in what settings do these activities take place; what limitations or constraints exist for them because of protocol, rules, standard operating procedures, and so forth. Such a focus allows for the possibility that the nature of the job may precipitate burnout and not just the nature of the person performing that job.

Indeed, this is the position that my research findings strongly support. Although personality does play some part in burnout, the bulk of the evidence I have examined is consistent with the view that burnout is best understood (and modified) in terms of situational sources of job-related, interpersonal stress. The phenomenon is so widespread, the people affected by it are so numerous, and their personalities and backgrounds are so varied, that it does not make sense to identify "bad people" as the cause for what is clearly an undesirable outcome.

Rather, we should be trying to identify and analyze the critical components of "bad" situations in which many good people function. Imagine investigating the personality of cucumbers to discover why they had turned into sour pickles without analyzing the vinegar barrels in which they had been submerged!

EXPLAINING SITUATIONAL STRESS IN PERSONAL TERMS

If burnout is more a product of bad situations than of bad people, then surely the individual in such a setting should recognize the situational forces out there and deflect the blame from inner self to outer environment. Not so.

The "Mea Culpa" Reaction

More often than not, people interpret their experience of burnout as reflecting some basic personality malfunction. The feeling that "something is wrong with me," "I am too weak or incompetent to handle this job," or "I have become a bad person" is pervasive enough to propel many people into some form of self-condemnation. Some seek therapy to understand their inadequacy, but probably more battle the problem with booze or rush it away with drugs. Even when they are able to acknowledge the situational stresses from a job demanding too much contact with too many others–"My work load is impossible"–they are still too ready to blame some flaw within themselves ("I should have been able to handle it," "I should have tried harder and put out more effort," and so on).

Why do we tend to have this strong bias toward blaming burnout on ourselves, rather than on features of the work situation? To begin with, much psychological research informs us that many people have a general tendency to overestimate the importance of personal factors, while simultaneously underestimating situational ones (a tendency that psychologists call "the fundamental attribution error").[13] For example, when someone states an opinion, we usually assume it expresses that person's true beliefs and rarely consider how much it is influenced by the other people who are present (as when an opinion is intended to please and flatter people or to shock and provoke them). We not only pay more attention to people than to the environment, we think in terms of individual differences between persons and have an extensive vocabulary of personality traits with which to characterize people. There is no comparable richness in our descriptors of the personalities of different situations.

For these and other reasons I will discuss later, we tend to overlook the contributions of the environment to people problems. We see someone behaving in a particular way because "he's that kind of person," and not because he is in a setting that elicits that behavior. Even when our own behavior is actually being determined by the situation we are in, we do not always recognize that fact, because we take the context for granted if we have been in it over a period of time. It is just the background, while the individual is the actor and main figure. For example, a teacher's attitude toward a pupil may have been affected by what other teachers had reported previously, but she may still believe that she arrived at her position (of agreeing with them) entirely on her own. In addition to this general tendency to underestimate the impact of situations on behavior, several unique elements in the caring relationship lead people to blame themselves for burnout.

First of all, the burnout syndrome appears to be a response to chronic, everyday stress (rather than to occasional crises). The emotional pressure of working closely with people is a constant part of the daily job routine. What changes over time is one's tolerance for this continual stress, a tolerance that gradually wears away under the never-ending onslaught of emotional tensions. As a result, when a caregiver begins to have problems in dealing with people, he or she has difficulty in identifying their situational cause. There is no immediate change in the work environment that corresponds with the noticeable change in his or her behavior. "This job has always been stressful, but I'm just starting to have troubles now–so the job can't be the reason for them." In fact, the stress of the job *is* the cause. However, since the job is a constant factor, while the person's problems vary over time, the person is unable to see a situational cause that coincides with the effect. Therefore, the obvious choice is between two possible causes, both person-centered: "The problems are caused either by me or by them."

We are more likely to attribute burnout to ourselves if we believe that our reaction is unique, and thus not shared by others. Such a belief results from the phenomenon of "pluralistic ignorance"–"Nobody knows the troubles I've seen because they all seem so happy, so I'll pretend to be happy too so nobody will suspect that I've seen troubles." People hide their true feelings and act as if everything were peachy keen and A-OK. When everybody puts on this mask of "I'm doing just fine" and fails to share his or her true reactions, then other suffering souls in the same boat are going to assume erroneously that they are alone in their distress. "It looks like *they* all know what they are doing–but *I* don't." This misinterpretation is strengthened when the individual who feels like a "sore thumb," a "weak link," or a "sob sister" in not being able to hack it works hard at not revealing this "deviant" response to others. Instead of self-disclosure what we see is displaced effort to display publicly the "I'm all right, Jack" facade. This process is poignantly illustrated by the experience of a former nurse in the Midwest:

> While we were in training, we were always being told to "be professional." No one ever said exactly what "professional" meant, or how to be that way, but I guess we all figured out that it meant being cool, calm, objec-

> tive–and not being easily rattled by things. But I *did* get rattled and upset at times–like the first time a patient died. And I would be feeling panicky and angry and sad, but I would be fighting any expression of those feelings because I knew they were *not* professional. Everyone else seemed to be handling things OK, which made me feel even worse–like a real failure and a weakling who wasn't cut out for this kind of work. And I didn't dare say anything to them, for fear they would find out how weak I was and would think badly of me. It wasn't until much later that I discovered that they were just as scared and lonely as I was, and afraid that I would think badly of them!

When people are working with others in the context of an institution, "administrative response" is another unrecognized factor that leads them to misperceive the cause of burnout as coming from within themselves. If difficulties arise in the delivery of care or service, administrators and supervisors are programmed to see the problem in terms of subordinates who are not performing their job adequately, rather than of shortcomings in the operational features of the institution itself. Because they assume that many of the hassles result from errors, faulty judgments, or laziness on the part of the employees, a major aspect of the job of administrators is directed toward getting employees to improve their job performance or getting better employees–the old "shape up or ship out" motivational advice. Thus, when employees complain to administrators about the emotional stress of their work, the typical person-oriented response is, "What's the matter, can't *you* take it?" Or, "What seems to be *your* problem?" In one stroke the administrator takes the institution off the hook and hangs the complainer on it instead. By having the blame laid squarely in the person's lap–"It must be something about *you* that is wrong, nobody else is dissatisfied or making problems"–a sense of alienation, failure, and self-hatred are fueled. "You're right, there must be something wrong with me." In *sotto voce:* "I wonder what that something could be?"

Putting the Blame on the Other Guy

The bias toward blaming people for burnout does not always mean that the person to be blamed is oneself. The fault may be attributed to the other person in the relationship. The burned-out teacher blames the students, the medical staff hold the patients responsible, the prison guards blame the inmates, parents say it's the kids' fault, social workers blame the clients, and on and on. "I'm burning out because of *them* (they're always complaining, they never learn, they're obnoxious, they're losers, and so on)." After we have pointed a damning finger at the other guys, our hostility and resentment toward them are less restrained. Once such prejudiced attitudes are translated into negative actions, it becomes easier to justify treating "those people" in less than humane ways ("Why should I be polite to someone like that?"). Over time, the callousness and cynicism of burnout come to full bloom–or rather, full withering.

Any difficulties that the other people may be experiencing in life are attributed to their inherent "defects" rather than to their current situation ("It's their own damn fault that they don't have enough money"). This response is known as *blaming the victim* and is related to the belief that people get what they deserve in this world (so if they don't have much, it's because they must not have deserved it).[14] Blaming the victim is even more likely to occur when the true causes of the victim's problems are not clearly identifiable. For example, the true cause of a family's poverty may be the social-economic-political structure of society, which discriminates against them in various ways. Such a pervasive, abstract, and complex cause cannot be easily pinpointed; it has no specific boundaries in time and space. There's nothing to hold on to, nothing that any person can do something about and observe some change taking place. When the situational cause is not clear or is embedded in a broad complex of factors, we are likely to hear conclusions like: "It can't be the situation—the problem is the people themselves."

Within various health and social service professions additional factors promote people-oriented explanations. Many professional staff see their clients or patients on an individual basis about their difficulties, rather than meeting with groups of people who share the same problem. This contact with separate individuals leads professionals to analyze the problem in terms unique to the person, locating its causes somewhere within him or her. When dealing with a series of single individuals, the helping professional tends to focus on what it is about each person that is causing his or her problem. This is true even when the series of individuals all have the same difficulties but are seen one at a time. What might happen if all of them were to appear en masse at the therapeutic doorstep, asking for help? There is little doubt that the professional would approach this apparent epidemic by investigating what is wrong with the situation they all are in.

> I once talked to a psychologist at a University Student Health Center about the problems of shyness and loneliness among the students. He said that this was indeed a source of difficulty for many students—that he saw several hundred of them with this problem over the course of the school year. When I asked how he treated this problem, he talked in terms of the individual student: his or her personality characteristics, family history, motivation to succeed, failure to risk taking the initiative, and so on. "These students come to your office on an individual basis, correct?" "Yes." "But what would have happened if a hundred of them appeared at once, saying they were shy and lonely?" "Then, of course, I would have to assume that something was happening on campus to make so many people feel that way. I'd call the dean or the dormitory adviser to find out what was up."

In many institutional settings the very structure of the records kept on each client or patient contributes further to this people-oriented bias. The forms to be filed typically ask for a trait characterization of the person—his or her problem, critical incidents, "beefs" or staff complaints, and other personal evaluations. Usually, there is no place in the report form for listing *circumstances* that elicited the reactions noted. For instance, a client's belligerence might be viewed differently in the context of her having had to wait several hours to see a staff person or having been given a runaround. There is not a space on the form for the client or patient to respond with his or her version of what appears to be "unprovoked" or "unjustified" action. Situational circumstances, if not ignored entirely or minimized, are honored at best with the status of excuses. And, of course, we do not accept an excuse as an explanation. Within the institution these records take on a historical "truth." They become the standard against which the actual person is measured when he or she reappears in the provider's office. These matters of record may bias the judgments that the provider will make in the face-to-face encounter. For example, if the file says the prisoner is a troublemaker, the guard may see him as making more trouble than he really is and thus as requiring more surveillance. Rebelling against this unnecessary surveillance helps fulfill the behavioral prophecy–he is a troublemaker. In this way, the written record both creates and maintains a focus on the individual person with problems, which enhances our tendency to find such a person at fault in situations where burnout occurs most often.

Whether the brunt of the blame is carried by the giver or the recipient of care, blaming either allows the contribution of the situation to burnout to be minimized or ignored. If the appropriate situational causes are not recognized or appreciated, we can be sure that attempted solutions for burnout will be misguided or incomplete. Therefore, a situational analysis is a major theme of this book.

In the next two chapters I will explore the major situational bases of burnout. First I will present the psychological dynamics of the involving interaction with people, and then I will investigate the nature of the work settings in which such interaction takes place. Next, I will consider what the individual brings to these situations, in terms of personal motives and personality traits that may increase vulnerability to burnout. Having analyzed the various sources of burnout, I will focus on its consequences and assess the deleterious effects it can have for the individual, for other people in the relationship, and for the relevant organization. The last three chapters will attempt to answer the question, "OK, so now we know what burnout is; what do we *do* about it?" Techniques for coping effectively with the syndrome as well as strategies for preventing it from happening in the first place will be presented in the hope that, if implemented, they can help reduce the increasing number of burnout casualties. By discovering how to lessen the psychological stresses of our jobs, as well as how to handle better those that remain, we are helping to reaffirm the human connection between all those who give help and those who need help.

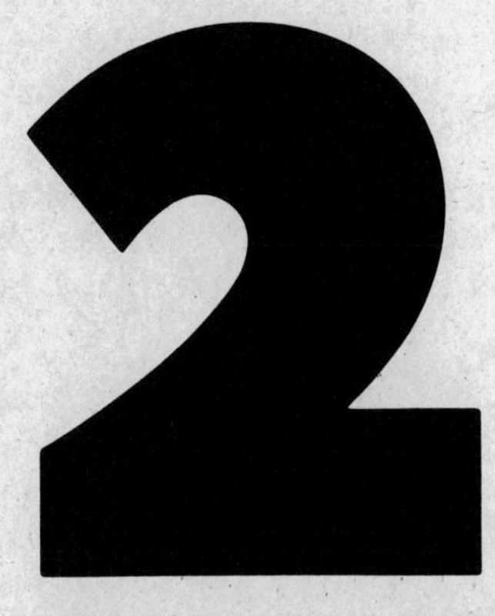

INVOLVEMENT WITH PEOPLE AS A SOURCE OF BURNOUT

Dear Abby:

My problem is my job. I am a bus driver in Tacoma, Wash. I can handle the traffic, but the people are driving me bananas. I've been driving a bus for four years now, and I don't know how I've lasted this long. Can you give me some information on becoming a shepherd? . . .

Fed Up[1]

Suppose you have patients, who, when you approach their bed, turn away with a growl on their face and swear at you. They may do that to everybody, but nevertheless it's hard on you. Suppose you have to give them medicines four times a day, and after the twenty-eighth time of them refusing their medicines—not talking, not saying anything, just looking terrible and swearing at you behind your back—you just really wonder with frustration if you can put up with much more of it. If you take it personally, then you'll feel that way. If you know that it's them, and how bad it must be at that point for them, then you don't feel that way. Most of the time you can handle it, but if you've got other things on your mind—well, it's very hard to do all the time.

Sylvia H., psychiatric nurse

Dealing with people can be very demanding. It takes a lot of energy to be calm in the midst of crises, to be patient in the face of frustrations, to be understanding and compassionate when surrounded by fear, pain, anger, or shame. While most people can find the energy to do it occasionally, and some people have the resources to do it often, it is, as Sylvia H. says, very hard to do all of the time. And yet, "all of the time" is the expectation we have of people workers.

Although we pay lip service to the idea that "we're all human," "everybody has an off day," and "everybody makes mistakes now and then," we do not think that way when someone falls short in his or her dealings with *us*. As the recipients of service or treatment, we are sensitized to the times when the provider has been unconcerned and has failed to do a good job. But we are often insensitive to our own role in that process—what we, as recipients, contribute toward the burnout of the provider or caregiver. We must keep in mind that it takes two to tango—that there are two participants in any helping or caring relationship, each of whom helps shape and direct the course of that contact. Each one contributes toward the emotional stress of the mutual involvement (often unintentionally), just as each one contributes to the rewards and satisfactions. For example, X is anxious and worried because Y is so upset and depressed, while Y is bothered by the inability of X to understand Y's problem. Both X and Y act and react to each other in an interrelated process that can escalate into a more intensely stressful situation. Thus, to understand the phenomenon of burnout, we must understand the nature of people's involvement with other people.

SEEING PEOPLE IN NEGATIVE TERMS

A virtual hallmark of the burnout syndrome is a shift in the individual's view of other people—a shift from positive and caring to negative and uncaring. People are viewed in more cynical and derogatory terms, and the caregiver may begin to develop a low opinion of their capabilities and their worth as human beings. "I can't believe some of the weirdos we get here," "they come out from under the rocks," and so forth. These negative views help underscore and exaggerate the differences between "us" and "them," a process that has been described as "moral evaluation."[2] Consider the reaction of Rick S., a school aide who tests children's vision:

> Sometimes we find vision problems that are clearly affecting the child's performance in school. So we contact the parents and explain the problem and tell them where to go to get corrective lenses or treatment. But what amazes me is how some of these parents do nothing—they don't bother to get glasses for their kid, no matter how often we call them, or help set up appointments with an eye doctor, or offer to take them to the doctor ourselves. They just nod their heads and say, "Oh yes, yes, I

> understand and I'll take care of it right away"—but they don't take care of it and their kid is still struggling in school because he can't see the blackboard clearly. Maybe they don't have enough money—but somehow I know that if it were *my* kid, it wouldn't matter how poor I was, because I would hock everything to get my kid those glasses so he wouldn't fail in school. No one would have to ask *me* twice about it—I'd be the first one in line to see the eye doctor.

Such negative viewpoints are not the exception, held by only a small minority of people. A review of research on professional helpers, such as therapists, counselors, teachers, and social workers found that they have a consistently more negative evaluation of the people they help than do the general public.[3] This was true even when the people being evaluated were perfectly normal and not experiencing any major difficulties. What happens if helpers do not have positive perceptions of the people they are supposed to help? They may not like these people very much, may not be really motivated to help them, and the help they do provide may be less than their best or sometimes only more than their worst. For these reasons it becomes important to find out why this negative bias occurs.

Ironically, the very structure of the helping relationship promotes and maintains a negative view of people. Four aspects of this relationship are especially critical: the focus on problems, the lack of positive feedback, the level of emotional stress, and the perceived possibility of change or improvement.

Focus on Problems

By definition, recipients in most helping relationships are people with problems. The reason they are seeking help is that they are sick, in trouble, failing, depressed, unable to care for themselves, or experiencing some other type of difficulty. This negative part of themselves and their life is what the professional helper sees and is most concerned about. What is good and healthy about them is given less attention or is even ignored, since it is less relevant to the problem under consideration. "We have to know what's wrong with people in order to help them with their problem—we don't need to worry about what's already all right." This selective focus on weaknesses and deficiencies, rather than strengths and assets, is illustrated in the case of a couple who went to a mental health clinic and were first asked to fill out a questionnaire:

> The real stopper came on page two with the question, "Which of these statements best describes you as a parent: too strict, too permissive, too cold, too affectionate?" The guilt of the parents is assumed; all the statements are negative; the only question is which one to choose. Not once in four pages of information-gathering were the parents asked, "What do you think you have done right for your child?" or "What do you think are your redeeming qualities as a parent?"[4]

Helpers ask only about negative information often in the belief that the cause of a problem is located in some other negative aspect of the person. In addition, the clients themselves sometimes deliberately withhold positive information from the helper because it might reduce the amount of funds or services that they could receive. An exclusive focus on people's problems is also more likely as the number of people increases. The more people the caregiver has to worry about, the less time and assistance any one of them can receive. Consequently, what little time exists is parceled out on only the most serious and urgent problems. Spending time on the positive aspects of clients' lives is a luxury that simply cannot be afforded. Helpers in such time-scarce, people-filled jobs will inevitably have an incomplete knowledge and understanding of any single recipient; in a sense, they cannot see the trees for the forest.

Moreover, in most helping relationships when the recipients' problems disappear, so do the recipients. Once people are healthy and functioning well they have no further need for a professional helper, and so that relationship is ended. From the caregiver's point of view, this reduces the opportunity to see people in good times as well as bad. Those who return to see the helper usually do so only because the problem has returned. As one counselor put it, "My successes go away, but my failures come back to haunt me." Because of this continuous and limited focus on people's problems and flaws, it is not surprising that professional helpers begin to develop a negative and rather cynical view of human nature. Not only are suckers born every minute, but helpless creeps are cloned each second in the view of some burned-out helpers.

Lack of Positive Feedback

Whenever we do something for people, we like to hear how well it turned out—did they like it or not, did it help, did it make any difference? This feedback not only tells us if we did a good job, but it lets us know whether our efforts were appreciated. Just like anyone else, professional helpers like to get this feedback. They need the same reinforcing strokes as ordinary folk do. However, for them feedback is either nonexistent or is almost exclusively negative. They don't hear much when things are going right, but they sure hear plenty when things are going wrong. They hear complaints or criticisms about the job they are doing, they may be blamed for not giving enough help, and in some instances they are the targets of hostile remarks or even threatening actions. Some of this negative feedback may be a justifiable response to errors they have made, but sometimes it is a deliberate strategy to speed up service. If the person complains enough, the helper will work faster to provide the help just to silence the complaints—the "squeaky wheel" gets greased. As one prisoner recently wrote to me: "If I make myself a big enough pain in the ass, with prisoner litigation suits, complaints to the press, organizing inmate strikes, then maybe they'll want to send me home sooner."

Helpers are also on the receiving end of some very strong emotions of anger, fear, and frustration. Although they are not the direct cause of the person's plight, they may symbolize those causes or at least the forces that are preventing the person from achieving a solution to his or her problem.

> In January 1975, the welfare offices in San Francisco were faced with rapidly growing numbers of people applying for public assistance. There were no additional staff to handle the applications, and consequently, people who were desperate and in need of immediate help had to wait for one or two weeks before being interviewed. In one office the following events occurred:
>
> - There was a bomb threat and the building had to be evacuated.
> - Two days later, a welfare worker was shoved to the floor by a client and struck in the head and back.
> - The following day, a client kicked through the glass door at the entrance to the building.
> - A few days after that, a worker who was spending her lunch hour issuing an emergency check to a client was jumped from behind and repeatedly struck.
> - A client made his way to the coffee shop on the fifth floor of the building and attempted to rob the cash register.
> - During the first two weeks of the month, two guards stationed on the first floor, near the entrance, decided they had had enough and quit.
>
> According to one intake worker, "Our clients are hostile and violent—the bullet holes in the ceiling are a constant reminder of this. We are not serving their needs, and their anxieties are now beyond anyone's control."[5]

Recipients who are all too ready to dish out negative feedback rarely give positive feedback, however minimal, for things that the provider does well. The provider's work is simply taken for granted. "So you solved this problem—so what? That's what you're being paid to do." "What do you mean, I should say thank you? Parents are *supposed* to be like that." If a caregiver's accomplishments are expected as part of the job, then there is no need to provide feedback except when things fall short of these expectations (and then, of course, the feedback is negative). Our society makes matters worse by setting very high standards for helpers, which are difficult to achieve and impossible to maintain over a long time. Helpers are expected *always* to be warm, giving, patient, and courteous, and *never* rude, abrupt, hostile, or cold. If the helper meets that standard, there is rarely applause or congratulations—"That's not so special, that's what we expect of you." But when the expectations are not met, there is more than enough criticism. It is a chronic no-win situation—either you lose or you get nothing.

> Police officers have more than their share of unpleasant contacts with people, whether they be criminals or victims of crime. I once asked a New York cop what were his pleasant encounters with the public. He thought for a moment, and then said, "Well, in the past few years, I've helped deliver five babies in emergency situations. Now that should be a happy occasion—a baby being born, and everything's turned out OK even though it looked kind of scary at first. But you know, not once did anyone ever say 'thank you'—not once! I don't ask for much, but it would have been nice to know that they were glad I was there."

Positive feedback may not be given because it does not occur to people to give it, or they forget, or they fail to act on good intentions ("I keep meaning to write a thank-you note, but . . ."). In other instances, positive feedback is not forthcoming because the people involved are unable to provide it.

> For example, caretakers of cancer patients sometimes feel that they get little or no supportive feedback from the patients. "Although this is understandable in view of the serious illnesses [the patients] face, it makes things particularly difficult on the staff when the patients die. Some expressed this by saying, 'What's the payoff in this work?' This problem was especially acute when caretakers felt that a patient had 'given up and died.' "[6]

The upshot of this bias toward accentuating the negative and eliminating the positive is people contact that is unpleasant and unrewarding. Over time, caregivers begin to feel negatively about the ungrateful people themselves. For those whose major motivation in entering a helping or teaching profession was to work with people, making their lives better, the lack of positive feedback or "strokes" from them is a particularly bitter pill to swallow. At some point, many decide to stop swallowing that distasteful medicine.

Level of Emotional Stress

If the nature of his or her contact with people is especially upsetting, depressing, or difficult, then the provider may develop more negative or even dehumanized perceptions of them. Imagine the stress of contact with people who engage in highly objectionable or taboo behavior (such as committing child rape, or smearing feces on the walls of the psychiatric ward). Or consider what it is like to work every day with people who are physically or verbally abusive toward you. For many individuals contact with someone who is dying (particularly when it is a child) is most difficult of all. Research has documented that having to inform a patient or patient's family of impending death is the experience that medical students find most threatening.[7]

In instances such as these the helper feels helpless–helpless to control, change, or cure. The frustration and anger produced by such helplessness may be expressed in either malice or aversion.[8] Malice or hostility may occur even though professional ethical standards prohibit it. Such reactions occur less often when the person cannot be considered "at fault" for the condition, as when a child has cancer. In that case the anger may be displaced onto other people, such as fellow staff members. Then it erupts in endless bickering and disputes over irrelevant or trivial matters. The expression of aversion, however, *is* directed at patients or clients, by avoiding contact with them and dealing with them as little as possible.

> The psychotherapist may experience aversion in relation to the child with cancer both directly and unconsciously. A promise to "drop by tomorrow" is forgotten. A schedule suddenly becomes "too crowded for an appointment this week." An adolescent who gripes, "I don't need any help," is permitted to withdraw emotionally instead of being engaged in dialogue.[9]

Although there is general agreement on certain types of personal contact that are especially stressful, there are also many individual reactions. What may be especially difficult or upsetting for one person will not be for someone else. For example, child protective service workers in one agency in the Southwest had very different opinions on what was the hardest situation for them to handle. One worker said that working with a family in which incest had occurred was the most emotionally stressful for him; another was more bothered working with children who were victims of neglect. Some clinical psychologists report that working with sociopaths is the most stressful for them, others point to the depressed client who "just sucks me of all my energy," and still others feel most frustrated by a weepy, clinging, overly dependent client. A psychiatric nurse in one West Coast hospital describes frankly how the stress of involvement with others can lead to devaluating them:

> *Joan R.:* I had a really great experience working in an outpatient department. It was very different, because you don't get into such an intense relationship. But in an inpatient setting, it can get really heavy. There's an incredible amount of emotion and frustration, and sometimes you deal with it by putting down the situation, but it's the patient who gets put down in the end. Let's say that there is a patient who's incredibly isolated and hostile at the same time–just a son of a bitch to work with and get involved with. You know they're hurting so bad, and you know they really, really need you, and yet they're consistently terrible to work with. Sometimes you can't help but feel, "Damn it, they want to be there, and they're fuckers, and let them stay there." You really put them down–"They're patients, they can stay there forever, but I'm going home."
>
> *Interviewer:* Do you leave?

Joan R.: Hell, yes. You know, it's the end of your day and you don't have to stay. Sometimes just out of frustration you say that.

Interviewer: How long would you feel that way?

Joan R.: Until I thought about it. You know if you've got that strong a feeling that there's a lot going on inside of you, and it's not just them.

So now the person with a problem develops a new problem—how to handle the helper's hostility.

Possibility of Change or Improvement

Our view of people is affected by their responsiveness to us. If they do *not* respond to us, as a helper or simply as a fellow human being, then we become prone to develop negative feelings about them. People who do not acknowledge our presence, do not provide feedback, or fail to follow our advice or guidance are "de-humanizing" us, and it becomes easier, in turn, to dehumanize them and hold negative attitudes about them. Staff members working with chronic schizophrenics in an outpatient setting or with severely retarded individuals have reported how frustrating the experience can be at times: "It's like talking to a wall—nothing comes back. I don't know if they've even heard me, much less understand what I'm saying. And you have to keep working on the same things over and over and over again—there's no change sometimes, no matter what you do."

As illustrated in this last comment, a person reacts not only to the lack of personal responsiveness in others, but to the lack of change or improvement in their condition. In spite of all efforts to make an appreciable difference in someone else's life, nothing happens—nothing has changed or gotten better as a result. To ward off feelings of personal failure and ineffectiveness, the helper may blame other people for their problems, by seeing them as inherently defective, unmotivated to change, bad, or weak. (This is an example of the tendency to blame people, rather than situations, that I discussed in Chapter 1.)

Related to the notion of lack of change is the distinction between chronic and acute problems. From the helper's point of view, chronic problems are the constant, seemingly endless ones. They do not change much over time, regardless of effort or resources expended. They may not be highly stressful problems to deal with, in and of themselves, but they are always there and never go away. In contrast, acute problems or "crises" may be more severe, but they are also less frequent and often clearly linked to a definite cause. In some ways, it is easier to know how to handle a crisis than to handle a chronic problem. Professional helpers are often well trained in crisis intervention but are less well equipped to deal repeatedly with the more mundane problems of people who won't go away and who don't show signs of improving. Both for professional helpers and "non-professional" caregivers, the chronic problems are more emotionally draining and more closely linked to burnout. Any parent can tell you that it is the continuous, never-ending, twenty-four-hours-a-day obligation of raising children that is most debilitating. As another example, burnout among high school teachers was found to be related to the *frequency* of conflicts and disagreements with students (and not their severity).[10]

> A vivid illustration of the chronic-acute distinction is provided by the volunteer staff of a suicide prevention center in California. Of all the incoming calls, very few are from people who are seriously considering suicide at that moment. Most are from the "chronics," who call one or more times a day, every day, for weeks on end. They may be people who are lonely or who have personal problems of some kind, but they don't seem to improve as a result of talking to the staff—they just keep calling. A new staff person who unknowingly gets a chronic caller may invest a lot of time and emotional energy in talking to the person, only to hang up and discover that he or she is the latest person to fall for the caller's "routine." "So you got George, huh? Welcome to the club! Did he feed you the same old line he's been doing for years? Don't worry, you'll hear it again."
>
> After a few experiences like this, the staff member is likely to feel "burned" and used by callers, will begin to dread answering the telephone, and may become more callous toward callers who are perceived as trying to con him or her. Although the staff are trained to handle calls from someone about to commit suicide, they rarely have the opportunity to put their training into effect. As one staff member, Marcia D., put it, "Sometimes I catch myself thinking, 'I wish a real suicide call would come in, so I could use all my skills and handle it successfully. It would be an exciting challenge, not like all this tedious, humdrum stuff.' And then I think, 'My God, what am I saying? I *want* someone to try and commit suicide? Just so I can be a hero?' It's awful, but sometimes I feel like that."

THE OTHER PERSON

The fact that a person needs something from you may be sufficient to motivate you to try to provide what is needed. However, the *kind* of person you are dealing with may influence what you provide, how well you do it, and even whether you will do it at all. Obviously, it is more pleasant and personally rewarding to be involved with someone who is likable than with someone who is a pain in the neck. In most of our personal relationships we choose who we want to be with—and we usually choose people who are interesting and fun to be with, people who make us feel good and who are similar to us in background, interests, and values. But in our work relationships, we do not always have that choice. We may be asked to teach, help, or care for someone we do not like. We might have to deal with someone who is obnoxious, who has opinions that we find offensive, who intimidates us, or who is a "wet blanket." We may have to work with people who are very different from us in terms of age, social class, ethnic background, education–differences that can lead us to perceive them as alien and "not like me."

That particular people are not likable to us may say as much about us as it does about them. The point is that this "likableness" can intrude, for better or for worse, on the helping relationship. Recipients who are likable may get good care and positive attention from providers, but those who are unlikable may get shortchanged by the staff.

> A study done in a California mental hospital found that psychiatric evaluations were closely linked to how much staff members liked the patients. Patients who were well liked were judged as less mentally ill and as improving in their condition. However, patients who were disliked were recommended for more drug medication. Staff members tried to avoid contact with these disliked patients and recommended them for transfers to other wards. They even tried to "get rid" of these patients by recommending them for discharge–in spite of the fact that they also judged these patients as more mentally ill![11]

Just about everybody has his or her own rogue's gallery of "good" and "bad" clients, patients, students, or whoever. Common among the "bad" ones are people who are constantly demanding more care and complaining that what they get is less than they deserve. Others fail to follow instructions on how to care for themselves or seem to foil every attempt to help them. Another "bad" group are people who expect instant cures or successes rather than advice, and who get impatient regarding treatment. People who feign problems and who may have a bottomless need for attention can also drive you crazy, as Jim J., a substitute teacher, points out:

> The more I taught, the more I sensed a common theme in all those requests for bathroom passes, pencil-sharpening permission and notebook paper: "Gimme some attention." . . . The negative-attention syndrome must be the curse of the teaching profession. Time and again, I encountered students who obviously had brought their hunger for attention (and their anger) to school. They scuffled in class, rapped books on desks, slammed cabinet drawers and threw punches across the aisles, to name some of the milder behaviors. Teachers are caught: they don't want to feed the negative behavior with screams and threats but can't teach effectively with the disruptions, either. As one elementary school coach told me, "They'll get you if you don't get them first."[12]

These "bad" people are the ones that usually require more time, effort, and attention from the provider (and often on issues irrelevant to the main concern) and who make it unpleasant to spend any time with them. Also, if their behavior is based on some unrecognized need for attention or resistance, the helper may not know whether to take their statements at face value. Is the request or complaint legitimate, or is it not? How should I respond to it? As an example of the difficulty here, consider the predicament of physicians with critically ill patients who ask that they not be kept alive by a respirator but be allowed to die. In some cases this may be a very legitimate and reasonable request for a quiet and dignified death. But other patients may say this to get their families to pay attention to them, or they may change their minds several times, making it unclear what their "true" request is. Consider another example of how the pattern of complaints by a patient may lead to the conclusion that he or she is "faking it."

> Mrs. A was an elderly patient with cancer of the breast. She was usually a cheerful and active patient. Following a disagreement with her physician, she began complaining about the medication. She moaned so loudly that she was heard in the hall and at the nurses' station. The staff showed some skepticism over the seriousness of her condition. One nurse summed up this feeling by indicating the selective nature of the patient's interaction, "She will respond least of all to daughters or family, only to doctors and nurses. She is probably on a kick. She may be sick but she has cried 'wolf' so many times!" The following day the patient said goodbye to the laboratory technician and told him that she did not expect to live over the weekend. Members of the staff again remarked that the patient was probably only trying to gain attention. There was no lessening of staff attention to her needs, however. Two days later Mrs. A died. The nurse supervisor remarked at the time that she was shocked at the patient's death. Other nurses expressed a measure of guilt because they had taken the patient's prediction of her own death so lightly.[13]

The extent to which they are manageable also distinguishes "good" from "bad" recipients. The person who is quiet, passive, does what he or she is told to do, and does not make trouble is more likely to be regarded as "good" because such a person is easy to take care of. In general, most of us have learned this passive-dependent role expected of patients or clients. We speak only in response to the helper's questions, we follow directions, we are still and unmoving during physical examinations, and we are reluctant to suggest an alternative approach to solving our problem ("The doctor knows best"). In this kind of situation the helper has knowledge, resources, and power, and the recipient does not. The helper gives, the recipient receives. This passive-dependent stance of recipients has several advantages for the helper. It can make the helper feel important and competent, since it is proof positive of being needed by people. It not only makes recipients more manageable, it allows them to be seen in more dispassionate, objective terms—as things to be processed, rather than as people. This makes it easier for the caregiver to avoid getting overly involved with recipients, but it can also set the stage for indifference toward them.

The passive-dependent role of recipients can be a double-edged sword for caregivers; although it can make contact with people easier, it also makes it more stressful. It reduces the recipient's own responsibility for helping in the treatment and places a tremendous burden of responsibility on the helper. The recipient's fate is in the helper's hands, and that fact can make any of the helper's decisions fraught with anxiety.

> For example, in California people who are dangerous to themselves or others can be hospitalized for seventy-two hours, against their will, by someone who has received special authority from the Health Department (pursuant to section 5150 of the Welfare and Institution Code). One psychiatric social worker who has this power to "5150" someone says, "It scares the hell out of me sometimes. You are taking over somebody else's life and making a decision for them—confining them against their will—and that's one hell of a responsibility!" Yet somebody has to take that action, as in the case of a young man who broke out all the windows of his apartment, put a hole in the door, complained of "evil spirits" coming out of the TV, asked where he could get a gun, and, earlier, had run out in the street completely naked and defecated on the sidewalk. He answered the door with a three-foot pole and struggled with police for five minutes before he could be restrained. "I get very upset by some of the 5150s I have to do," said the worker on this case, "especially when you see a person yelling and screaming and crying and really, really hurting."[14]

The dependent recipient's problems may be more emotionally overwhelming for the helper, particularly when some of them are caused by the helper's actions (as when treatment for one medical problem leads to development of another). In addition, the dependent recipient often clings to the helper for constant guidance and never seems to go away. When caregivers complain about people who "cannot stand on their own two feet," who call regularly about any problem no matter how trivial, and who cannot do anything on their own without specific directions, they may not realize that the problem is the recipients' passivity and dependence, which they themselves may have done much to encourage.

According to the argument presented in transactional analysis, helpers get overwhelmed by passive-dependent clients because they set up a relationship between themselves as Rescuers and the clients as Victims (rather than an equalitarian relationship). This process is illustrated by Claude Steiner's description of a therapist working with an alcoholic:

> Without any assurance of interest and willingness to participate from the alcoholic, he begins to act in the role of a Rescuer in which he does more than half of the work because the alcoholic has not really manifested any interest in stopping drinking or doing anything at all other than maybe coming to therapy sessions. The alcoholic "makes progress" for a while, but eventually, just when everybody thinks he is really getting better, he goes back to drinking. Part of his reason is often a gesture of resentment and a retaliation to the therapist's one-up stance. This is an instance of the Victim turning Persecutor as the Rescuer turns Victim. After the alcoholic

> persecutes the therapist by his "failure," laced possibly with midnight calls and excessive demands for help, the therapist switches to the role of Persecutor and begins to act in vindictive ways. He may begin to think of him as a "schizophrenic," may discount him, be angry with him because he is no longer being a good little Victim but is being instead a bad little Victim. At this point, the Rescuer has turned into Persecutor and the alcoholic is back in the Victim position.[15]

THE RULES OF THE GAME

Burnout can be affected by the sorts of rules that govern the contact between provider and recipient. These rules, which determine what is said and done and what is not, have the potential to increase the emotional stress of the helping relationship. Many are explicit, formally stated guidelines of the relevant institution (such as a school, welfare agency, or hospital), and I shall discuss them in Chapter 3. Other rules are implicit, unstated ones that operate when a giver and a receiver get together.

The most obvious of these implicit rules is the "etiquette" of appropriate, nonemotional behavior in a helping relationship. Such etiquette requires that recipients be passive, dependent, and quiet individuals who are seen but not heard and who don't make waves. The etiquette for helpers is that they are always kind, caring, calm, patient, and respectful toward others. These implicit rules can be so constraining that the people on both sides feel upset and dissatisfied with the relationship. Recipients feel demeaned and powerless, while caregivers feel artificial in their saintlike pose. Providers also feel under pressure to be different from their normal selves and to bottle up their true feelings. We sometimes keep a lid on our emotions because they are inappropriate or nonprofessional (as when a probation officer wants to yell back at a belligerent client but smiles and "bites his tongue" instead). In other cases, the lid is used to keep our own feelings from becoming overwhelming. For example, a routinized, stereotyped response to people helps make a painful job easier—as when a social worker has to tell a client that she cannot help further with the problem. Sometimes the helper must keep information secret—as when a dying patient wishes to "protect" her family from the news, or vice versa. This conspiracy of silence requires a constant vigilance not to let such information slip out either in words or in emotional expression. Emotions may also be hidden because they are apt to be judged as a sign of weakness, indecision, or incompetence. However, as one surgeon points out, there are costs attached to this professional rule of nonemotionality:

> Frequently we have difficulty in expressing our feelings to the patient. Early in our career, physicians learn to control the outward manifestations of emotions. Personal problems, fear, anger all are cloaked by the profes-

> sional manner. It would not be well for the patient to see our emotional status of the moment mirrored in our faces. We also learn that our compassion must be blunted so as not to suffer too much with our patients or we too would soon become ill. Thus has arisen the myth that we really don't care.[16]

When there is an emergency people act according to a different set of social rules than if the problem is a routine one. They act more quickly, they drop everything else to handle this top-priority problem, they give it their full attention, and they continue to follow up on it until the emergency has been resolved. Often everyone is more emotional—anxious, worried, fearful—than if the problem is one they have faced frequently. The difference between what constitutes a routine problem and an emergency is a source of chronic tension between a professional helper and a recipient. What is an emergency to the recipient is often routine to the helper, precisely because the helper *has* seen the problem a hundred times. Indeed, the choice of a helper is often made on the basis of his or her past experience with this particular problem. The helper is an expert, the sufferer a novice in dealing with the matter at hand. What this means, however, is that helper and recipient will be approaching the same situation with very different rules and expectations, and this can cause irritation, resentment, and frustration on both sides. The recipient may feel upset and angry by the seemingly casual and indifferent response to an important and all-consuming personal event. From the other side, the helper may get irritated by the recipient's exaggerations of the problem, making it out to be more serious than it really is. We see this antagonism in the continual disagreement between doctors and patients over diagnosis of the common cold. Each patient feels his or her cold is unique, with a set of symptoms suggesting a more serious illness (flu, pneumonia, perhaps the start of the black plague). From the doctor's perspective, this cold is no different from all other colds and requires no special treatment beyond the standard two aspirins, fluids, and rest. The patient, however, may not react kindly to this standard prescription, because it suggests that the doctor is not taking a special problem seriously but is treating this "uncommon" malady in common terms.

The routine versus emergency difference in perceptions is one example of a mismatch of expectations about the helping relationship. There may also be a mismatch regarding the goals of the relationship. The provider has a certain goal in mind and some ideas about what will take place to achieve it. The recipient, however, may have a different goal and different ideas about what is going to happen. This lack of agreement is often unrecognized by the two participants, because they usually do not make their assumptions explicit. Thus, each one enters into a helping relationship thinking that the other person shares the same expectations, when in fact they disagree.

> A client who comes to a legal services attorney may be experiencing many problems in her life and wanting help. She expects that the attorney will

> provide that help for all her problems (financial, emotional, and so on), while he expects to handle only those that involve clear legal issues. The dilemma that she wants to talk about most may not be the one he can do something about. He asks for information which he considers necessary for the case, but she resists giving it since she considers it an unwarranted invasion of her privacy. This clash of expectations can generate a great deal of friction and animosity between attorney and client. Furthermore, when the relationship has ended, the client is likely to feel cheated and frustrated at getting only a bare minimum of the aid she desired, while the attorney will feel that even doing his best is not good enough, since the client has continuous demands that never seem to be fulfilled.

This mismatch of expectations can cause problems in any sort of personal relationship, not just a helping one. Many couples who live together have "covenants," with each person expecting certain things and willing to give certain things to the relationship, and each one assuming that the other has agreed to this (when in fact the other has not). For example,

> Bill believes, only partly consciously, that if he answers certain of Lucille's needs as he perceives them, it is then understood between them that she, in turn, will fill his needs—which he has failed to express to her. Lucille has only a vague idea of what Bill expects of her. . . . But there is much more that Lucille has never thought about—and quite a bit that Bill has never thought about, either.[17]

Within the business world there may be a clash between people's ideas on how to be a leader. The woman executive who is agreeable and pleasant and who makes decisions in a democratic way may be judged as weak and may encounter resentment or resistance from people who believe an authoritative, "masculine" approach is needed to exercise power. In all of these situations there is the potential for personal conflict and emotional stress, because the participants are playing the same game by different rules.

IT COULD BE ME

THE ANATOMY LESSON[18]

October.
On eight stainless steel tables eight long packages lay
Each shrouded in green toweling; each wrapped in
Clear plastic.

We unwrap our gifts with care
And as we lift the covers
My students are probably thinking
Grandpa or Grandma,
Uncle Max or Aunt Sadie.

I remember my father, wasted by cancer.
The last time I saw him he didn't see me,
His face dull silver against white sheets.

I try not to see my mother.
So many of her friends are here.

For a moment
I see myself.

All through the winter I'm enthralled.
Captured, bound, enfolded.
Awake, asleep, my thoughts shuttle back and forth
Weaving a tangled plexus of science and sentiment.

Day by night and night by day
These bodies surrender their secrets.

Day by night and night by day
These bodies tug at my lab coat and whisper,
"Live."

George J. Fruhman
Albert Einstein College of Medicine

Contact with a troubled human being will always be more emotionally stressful if the trouble has personal relevance to the helper. When the person's plight resembles your own past experience, it brings back unpleasant memories or unresolved feelings. Or the person may be experiencing something that is certain to happen to you as well, such as death, and this may arouse strong fears and anxieties. One way to handle these personal feelings is by distancing oneself from the person who is "causing" them, thereby adding a layer to the callous detachment of burnout.

> Susan T., a poverty lawyer, was visited by a female client just before Christmas. While discussing her problems, the woman complained about the fact that she was so poor that she was not going to be able to get any Christmas presents for her children. Susan T. was a young mother herself and knew the special importance of Christmas for kids, and so she might have been particularly sympathetic to the woman's dilemma. Instead, she found herself yelling at the woman, "So go rob Macy's if you want presents for your kids! And don't come back to see me unless you get caught and need to be defended in court!" Afterward, in thinking about the incident, Susan T. realized she had burned out.

When people feel "it could be me," they may find it easier to empathize with the other person. They may be able to see things from the other's perspective and gain some insight into the problem. They can also share in the other person's feelings and understand the emotional turmoil he or she is going through. To have this personal experience of someone else's problem is sometimes held up as a necessity for a good helping relationship. Indeed, it is the argument for using role playing to gain experiential knowledge of the other. "You can't know what it's like until you've been there." Former alcoholics or drug abusers are hired to counsel current ones, and in the documentary "Scared Straight," adult criminals are seen working to prevent juvenile offenders from continuing a life-style that will lead the youth to become like them.

While there are certain advantages to having empathy for others, there are also some potential drawbacks. A person can overidentify with someone else's plight and add those feelings to his or her own, thus taking on an enormous emotional burden. Emotional closeness may bias perceptions and influence judgments in ways that are more detrimental than helpful. Objectivity may be lost just when a clear head is needed.

The problem here may lie with what we mean by *empathy.* Although most definitions refer to the ability to "get inside" another person, some describe an intellectual role taking while others describe an emotional sharing. In the first case the individual *sees* things from the other person's perspective, while in the second he or she *feels* the other person's emotions. In a helping relationship the ideal may be the intellectual understanding but not the emotional involvement—that is, to understand the person's viewpoints on the problem but not to take on his or her feelings of fear, anger, shame, and so on. "I see where you're coming from, but your pain is not going to be mine."

However, separating out the two kinds of empathy is easier said than done. For most people, the two go together and are not thought of as distinct. It is difficult to get into a person's head without getting tangled up in the person's feelings as well. There is rarely good training for professional helpers in this regard, and too often they take the direction to "be empathic" to mean "experience the other person's feelings" rather than "see things from the other person's point of view." A positive value is often placed on "feeling what the other person feels," without considering that such feelings can produce the emotional exhaustion of burnout when experienced over and over, week in and week out, with a variety of people. Also, this advice ignores the fact that one can care and be genuinely concerned about another individual without experiencing emotional empathy.

GETTING TOO CLOSE FOR COMFORT

Contact with people can be especially stressful if the individual gets too highly involved at a personal level. The helper may take on someone's problem as a special cause or may become close friends with a client. Whatever happens to that person then becomes the helper's special burden as well. If the other person makes hostile comments, the helper may take them personally rather than seeing them as part of the larger problem. According to Sam L., a psychiatric technician in a mental hospital:

> If someone on the outside were to hit me, I would get really angry and hit them back. But I try not to get angry when a patient hits me because it's a different situation. I try to remember that the patients who strike out are not really angry at me—they're striking out in fear or they're so out of it that they don't even know what they are doing. Sometimes a patient is striking out at the devil. So, at the moment, I happen to look like the devil, but it's not me personally that he's striking out at—so I try not to get angry at that.

Getting overly involved with people also occurs when those people satisfy some personal needs—such as a need for attention or recognition or appreciation of some sort. A teacher who gets very upset when a class does not give him its undivided attention may not be reacting so much to the lack of order as to the implied lack of respect or recognition of his skill and authority. A therapist may get impatient with a client's resistance in therapy because it challenges her sense of expertise. A nurse may get emotionally entangled with an elderly patient whose frustrating dependence on her is actually a boost to her self-esteem (an example of the double-edged sword mentioned earlier):

> A specific kind of patient . . . upsets me—that's the patient who says things to you like: "When you're not here, I'm so lost I don't know what to do." or "Walk down the hall with me; I can't go by myself." or "Who will take care of me if you go away?"
>
> It's not flattering to me; sometimes patients like this torture me on my day off, because they are angry and hurt when you leave, and you can't help but worry about how they'll be without you. . . . They make you feel like a mother; and when you go away, it's like a mother abandoning her children. . . . I do know that [the patient] doesn't fall apart when I'm not here; yet I do feel guilty when I leave her for my day off. . . . And that's not logical . . . these other nurses are good professionals. They do their job, and I know it—yet I act as if I don't. When I feel guilty and worried about her, I'm acting as if what she says is true—that I'm the only one who really helps her. And I guess it's because, without my realizing it, I did feel that her need for me proved what a good nurse I am.[19]

In Freudian psychoanalysis, *countertransference* refers to the personal reactions a therapist may have about his or her patient. The patient may be liked or disliked because of a perceived similarity with some significant person in the therapist's life. Or the patient may be fulfilling some unconscious needs of the therapist. More than most other helping professionals, psychoanalysts are explicitly told to watch for signs of countertransference in their therapeutic relationships and to deal with these feelings when they occur.

Whatever the reason for getting overly involved with people, being so close can be a problem when the relationship comes to an end. For professional helpers there will always be a termination point—the client gets better or simply stops coming or fails to respond to the help. And that termination can be emotionally devastating for those who are too closely involved. As one psychiatrist put it, "You invest so much in your clients—you work so hard for them and give so much of yourself—and then they go away. It can really be a crusher." In some cases, it is the helper who "goes away," not the recipient—but the trauma of termination is still great.

> Attorneys and their investigative staff who handle prison litigation sometimes find themselves getting deeply involved with their prisoner-clients. In part, this is a result of their own personal philosophy and dedication to the cause, but it also develops in response to the prisoners' tremendous needs for attention and human contact. The professional relationship may be supplanted by strong bonds of friendship or even romantic attachment. However, the personal needs of the prisoners are sometimes so great that the legal staff can never satisfy them, no matter how much extra work or how many special favors they do. Their sincerity and their credibility are continually being tested by the prisoners, who are quick to note when things fall short of expectations. Once the attorneys no longer represent the prisoners this termination of a professional relationship may be interpreted by the prisoners as a personal rejection. In the tragic case of Faye Stender, who had done more prison work than almost anyone else, her exit from prison litigation was viewed as a betrayal by the former inmate who tried to kill her.

As should be clear by now, the close encounters between provider and recipient play a central role in the development of burnout. However, our understanding of burnout will be incomplete if we focus only on the two people in the helping relationship. This relationship does not exist in a vacuum but takes place in a broader context, often an organizational one. It is shaped and influenced by that context in many important ways, as we shall see in the next chapter.

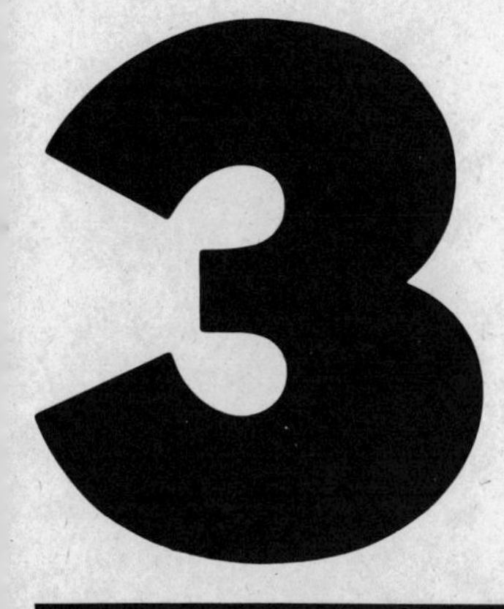

THE JOB SETTING AS A SOURCE OF BURNOUT

At Denver's Adams City High School, William Van Buskirk smoothed crisis after crisis—walkouts by political radicals, riots by angry chicanos, even gunplay in the halls—while maintaining an admirable educational program. His efforts won him a nomination by local educators in 1975 as one of Colorado's outstanding principals. But Van Buskirk paid a heavy price. He worked seven days and five nights a week until he grew exhausted physically and emotionally; he also ended up in divorce court. After eight years in that job, Van Buskirk quit to open a less taxing consulting firm. . . . "The teachers think you should control every one of the 1,800 kids," says Van Buskirk. "Parents expect you to make the halls safe and their kids normal in every way. When a teacher isn't dynamic, productive and well prepared, the board of education orders the principal to make him into a great teacher." . . . You're supposed to be a miracle worker," he says of his old position, "but nobody offers to help the principal on his job. I felt alone."[1]

Imagine the scene in a hospital emergency room: a young doctor in white confronts his patient—a young woman with slitted eyes and slurred speech. She has taken a handful of sleeping pills—a suicide gesture, a very common

> episode. Her boyfriend is standing by looking perplexed. . . . Imagine that the time is 3:30 in the morning and the intern has been working since 7:30 the previous morning. Remember that he knows he will be on duty until 5 or 6 that night, and that his routine has been repeating itself every other night for more than a month . . . now ponder the emotional response that the intern . . . might be experiencing while staring down at the young woman as she pleads for "Johnny." Empathy? On TV, yes. From your easy chair, yes. In real life? Anger! The intern is numbed by fatigue. For him, rationality may be impossible. His judgment is in flux. The patient becomes a problem to be solved—an assignment to be checked off. With misdirected hostility, the intern may well vent his frustrations on the patient.[2]

The contact between provider and recipient often occurs in the context of a formal institution, such as a school, hospital, or welfare agency. The provider is usually a trained professional, hired to deliver a particular service to people who are (at least initially) strangers. Many elements of this job situation define the nature of the care or service that is ultimately delivered—what kind, how much, when, for how long, and to what end. The resources that are available to the provider, the constraints that are placed on him or her, and the goals that are established are largely determined by the institution and not by the individual provider. Moreover, the relationships among people on the job—between provider and recipient, between co-workers, between staff and management—are shaped by the structure of the job setting. To the extent that job characteristics can either promote or reduce emotional stress, they become an important factor in the burnout syndrome.

In some cases the entire job is defined as "dirty work"—necessary work that is highly distasteful, unpleasant, or upsetting.[3] Society expects and demands that such work be done but often places a certain stigma on those who do it or fails to give them support or recognition for it. This makes the job doubly stressful and promotes the possibility of burnout. Human service professionals who do "dirty work" include prison guards, mental hospital staff, morticians, or psychiatric emergency teams ("the guys in the white coats who come to take you away"). Police, fire fighters, and other rescue workers are the ones called on to do the "dirty work" of handling disasters and cleaning up the human mess:

> In September 1978, an airliner collided with a small plane and crashed into a San Diego neighborhood in an accident that claimed 144 lives. Emergency personnel were confronted with a scene of horrifying human carnage, since parts of bodies were strewn everywhere. The trauma of working in this situation was so severe that many of the workers suffered from nightmares or insomnia, developed psychosomatic symptoms, or had anxiety attacks. About one hundred of them sought psychological treatment in an effort to cope with the overwhelming and sickening feelings aroused by their direct contact with the tragedy.

Many different job settings that are burnout-prone have one thing in common—overload. Whether it be emotional or physical, the burden that exceeds the person's ability to handle it is the epitome of what we mean by *stress.* Too much information is pouring in, too many demands are being made, and it is all occurring too fast for the person to keep up with it. For the professional helper overload translates into too many people and too little time to adequately serve their needs—a situation ripe for burnout. Such a situation exists in the work of service and claims representatives in Social Security offices, who spend most of their time in direct contact with the public. They can do a fine job and even enjoy it when they "service" twenty or thirty clients a day. When the number of people they see daily rises to forty or more, the telltale signs of burnout show up—emotional exhaustion, more negative feelings about the public, and a reduced sense of personal accomplishment.[4] Bill W., a West Coast welfare worker, expressed it this way: "There are just so many people, you cannot afford to sympathize with them all. If I only had fifty clients, I might be able to help them individually. But with three hundred clients in my case load, I'm lucky if I can see that they all get their checks."

When the case load is large the contact between helper and recipient is minimized in several ways. Less time is spent together, fewer services are provided, and there is little or no follow-up. Not only does the *quantity* of the contact change, but the *quality* does too. The helper develops a selective focus on problems in the person's life, since there is no time to "waste" on things that are already OK. This focus on problems promotes a negative view of the other person.

> In a study of staff in day-care centers, Ayala Pines and I found that burnout increased as the ratio of children to staff increased. With more children, a staff member spent more of his or her time handling immediate problems—breaking up fights, putting an end to teasing, cleaning up messes, comforting unhappy kids, treating bloody noses or scrapes, and so on. There was little "free" time to spend reading stories, playing games, or doing some other positive activities—any kid who was doing fine was left alone. As might be expected, these staff developed more negative attitudes about children, and when vacation time arrived, they wanted to get as far away from children as possible.[5]

The emotional strain of dealing with so many people may lead the provider to pull back psychologically and get less involved with each of them. The worker avoids physical contact by standing farther away from the other person or avoiding contact that makes a personal connection. A social worker says, "I don't look in the waiting room if I can help it. I don't like to see all that. I look at the name on my door, call it out, and head back into my office. I can handle them one at a time."[6] Other helpers may busy themselves with another task even while talking to the recipient, or keep one hand on the doorknob during an interview (a silent signal to "hurry up and get out of here"). Impersonal statements, superficial generalities, and form letters replace more personal communications. Psychological withdrawal is also evident in avoidance of certain tasks ("it's not my job") and hiding behind rules (the "petty bureaucrat" we saw in Chapter 1). Perhaps less obvious as a withdrawal response is doing a poor job, since this tactic ensures that fewer major problems will be referred your way. Ironically, if you do a good job in handling a particular problem, you usually get "rewarded" by getting more of them to handle. With such rewards, who needs punishment?

Thus, when there are too many people to serve, the helper develops both a quick and impersonal method of dealing with them. Not surprisingly, the quality of the care or service may deteriorate. We see this situation in many legal services offices.

> It is not unusual for a legal services attorney to be handling between 750 and 1,000 cases per year, and a substantial proportion have an even higher caseload. In contrast, an attorney in private practice rarely handles more than 500 cases per year. Faced with such an overwhelming number of clients, the legal services attorney has little time for pre-trial research and preparation. As might be expected, the result is dissatisfaction for the client as well as for the attorney. "We try a lot of cases by the seat of our pants—interviewing the client as we go into the courtroom, that sort of thing," one attorney observed. Given such pressures, the legal services attorney develops a rapid, emotionally detached method of dealing with clients. Key characteristics are used to define a specific set of "types." The "typing" or "slotting" procedure is at the heart of the assembly-line mentality that occurs in legal services offices, since it allows the attorney to apply formula solutions and to minimize personal involvement. This depersonalization is even more likely given the high level of repetition in most legal aid cases.[7]

Although emotional detachment is commonly used to cope with the crush of humanity, it is not the only response. Some helpers may get so overwhelmed by the press of people who need something, want something, and are always taking something from them, that they may lash out at the people themselves. They get irritated and frustrated by the endless stream of individuals, get angry at them and blame them for their own troubles, and sometimes just tell them to "go away, leave me alone, I can't give any more."

> Toward the end of the movie, *Jesus Christ Superstar,* an exhausted Jesus leans against a pillar of the temple following his confrontation with Jerusalem's money lenders. People surround him: old and young, well-dressed and shabby. They grasp at his clothes and at his hands, begging to

> be healed. "You're pressing too closely," Jesus mutters wearily. "There are too many of you and too little of me." Then with panic in his voice he cries: "Heal yourselves! Heal yourselves!"[8]

OUT OF CONTROL

Burnout is high when people lack a sense of control over the care they are providing. This lack of control can stem from being told by superiors exactly what to do, when to do it, and how, with no leeway to do it differently (even when the old formula is not working in some new situation). It can be a consequence of having no direct input on policy decisions that affect one's job. It can arise when a person has no opportunity to get away from a stressful situation or is given more responsibility than he or she can handle. Whatever the reason for the lack of autonomy, not perceiving control over important outcomes in one's job adds to the emotional strain of the helping relationship. Furthermore, this helplessness will not only make the helper feel more frustrated and angry, but will also promote feelings of failure and ineffectiveness.

Helpers can be "trapped" in their helping role by institutional rules that determine what their job will be. Such rules or job descriptions may force them to operate in situations that are very difficult or upsetting. Who wants to be the social worker assigned to a desk on the "front lines," telling clients why their checks are late? "Sorry for the administrative inconvenience–I hope getting your money next week won't be a hardship." The worker's contact with clients is bound to be unpleasant, and yet there is nothing the worker can do either to alleviate the problem or to escape from it. In some cases the job involves a necessary but unpopular task (another form of "dirty work"), designed to guarantee unpleasant encounters between people. One job that fits this category is collections–asking people to pay their bills–as illustrated in this woman's account:

> I'm called a patients' representative. My job is to admit them into the hospital. I'm the first one they see when they walk in the door and the last one to see when they leave. When they get their bills in the mail, they think of me. . . . When you ask for money first thing he comes in, it tends to upset the patient sometimes, unless you put it in a way that they're most grateful. I find the best way to do that, without myself being yelled at and called names, is to charm the patient and they calm down. "Are you aware what your benefits are? Do you have the means to pay the other fifty dollars a day?" They think you're informing them rather than demanding money. But you are demanding money. . . . If you owe me money, I can't ignore that fact. You may be sick and dying and I like you a lot and you make me cry and all that, I still got to go in and talk to you about your bill. That's what's hard."[9]

People may feel they lack control over their work because they have no voice or "say" in formulating the policies that affect their job. A common complaint among a variety of people workers is, "Somebody else makes the decisions, but *I* am the one who actually has to carry them out and do the shit work." If the policy decision is an unpopular one, the provider is the person on the firing line who takes the brunt of the criticism from recipients, even though he or she had no part in making the decision. In some public service institutions, such as the Social Security Administration, ever-changing rules and regulations are a consequence of the tide of new laws passed regularly by Congress. Not only do the Social Security employees have no input into these changes, but they are expected to implement them effectively and immediately even if the new rules are ambiguous, vague, arbitrary, and difficult to explain to clients.

Helpers can also feel trapped when the job does not allow them to take temporary breaks from stressful contact with people. They are on the spot, with no one else to share the work or help them out. How can they leave the recipient without feeling some guilt in doing so? Mothers with small children and no close friends or family nearby find themselves in this position; so may ministers counseling troubled parishioners. In more formal institutions this psychological "entrapment" can be a consequence of job specialization, in which helpers are required to provide care or service *all* the time, rather than having the opportunity to vary it with other, less stressful types of work. The more hours of direct, unrelieved contact with people, the greater the risk of burnout.

Feeling trapped can also arise from physical and economic limitations on changing jobs. The current job may be the best one available in the area where the helper wants to live or where the helper's spouse also has work. Or it may be the only job available in that particular profession because of cutbacks in funding services. Moreover, people may get locked into a job because they cannot afford to give up the benefits associated with it. Brian K., a high school teacher in a rural area of the eastern United States, puts it this way:

> Teaching tenure is an important benefit of this profession, designed to ensure job security for life. But it is also an alluring trap. One experienced teacher told me when I first began teaching, "If you are ever going to leave teaching, be sure to do it *before* you get tenure because it will be very hard to leave afterward." You can get trapped by the security the system gives, a lifetime security that keeps you teaching long after you've burned out.

CO-WORKERS: FRIENDS OR FOES?

Dealing with people on the job does not mean simply dealing with recipients. Co-workers, supervisors, and administrators are also significant people in the job setting, and the professional provider needs emotional energy and resources to relate to them as well. Sometimes these relationships can be even more stressful than the contact with clients or patients. According to Marie R., a young ex-teacher from the Northwest, "I really loved working with kids—that was the best part of the job, in fact. But I got turned off by the other teachers—I was always arguing with them, and some of my teaching innovations would get shot down by them for no good reason. And as for the principal—well, forget it."

Troubles in relating to one's peers, or co-workers on the job, can contribute to burnout in two ways. First of all, they are another source of emotional stress that adds to the development of emotional exhaustion and negative feelings about people. Second, they rob the individual of a very valuable resource for coping with and preventing burnout. As we shall see in Chapters 7 and 8, supportive relationships with one's peers can help stave off burnout in a variety of ways. If providers are put off by their peers, then they lack people to whom they can turn for help, comfort, advice, praise, or just a friendly pat on the back. They are alienated and alone in their battle against burnout, and that does not bode well for a successful outcome.

Some job settings seem designed to promote conflict between co-workers rather than cooperation. Co-workers may find themselves in competition with each other for favored positions, recognition, bonuses, and promotions. If this is the case, one-upmanship, backbiting, and put-downs are the order of the day. People are concerned about "me first" and may try to look good by making their peers look bad. Obviously, there are few attempts to help "the other guys" since there are no rewards for doing so and the helper only gets left behind as they move up. Furthermore, people are unwilling to ask for help or share their feelings, since doing so is often interpreted as a sign of incompetence or weakness. It may be used against them later on when a promotion report notes a lack of independence and overemotionality "in co-worker comments on the candidate." The lack of trust that exists in such job settings puts invisible walls between potential allies.

Peer conflict may also reflect displaced anger and frustration, as I suggested in Chapter 2. If providers cannot deal directly with the feelings aroused by their work with recipients, they may find other targets on which to vent their spleen. Thus, co-workers may engage in constant bickering and infighting, pick arguments with each other, and make mountains out of the molehills of trivial issues. Such interstaff hostility has resulted in instances where co-workers stop speaking to each other, even when they are supposedly part of a team effort.

> In one institution for severely retarded children the staff expressed positive attitudes toward the children even though acknowledging how difficult and challenging the contact with them could be. The staff also reported good relations with the children's parents. However, there was so much animosity and friction between the staff themselves that the staff members on each *hall* refused to get along with those on the other halls. They were warring teams under the same roof, and their hostility seemed far out of proportion to any actual disagreements.

A lack of rapport between co-workers can occur when they are members of different helping professions working together in a larger institution. One professional group may not think highly of another, and this can lead to invidious comparisons, professional put-downs, and even interference with one another's work. Different professions may see each other as rivals (for power or prestige), or they may simply lack knowledge and understanding of the other group's contributions and accomplishments. An example is the situation facing school counselors:

> An additional condition which makes it difficult for the counselor to maintain his helping position includes a deficiency in colleague support and a lack of understanding of counseling on the part of other school personnel. Counselors in schools are far outnumbered by teachers and administrators who may be suspicious or even hostile toward counseling. The psychological effects of being in a professional minority or of being misunderstood can lead one to question his own beliefs and practices.[10]

Distrust and distance between helpers can be fostered when the institutional administration discourages them from getting together. This happens when staff meetings or informal gatherings are seen as a "waste of time" or a sign of shirking professional responsibilities. Staff who seek support from their peers may be made to feel selfish, weak, lazy, or incompetent.

> The nurses on a ward for terminal cancer patients felt that the emotional strain of their work was so great that they needed some time each week for themselves—to talk over their experiences, get emotional support, and help each other when things got rough. They made a formal request for such a meeting, but the idea was pooh-poohed by the physicians and hospital director, who all felt that it would simply be an excuse for the nurses not to do their "real work" but to engage in "idle chitchat."

Peer relations also break down when a person voluntarily isolates him- or herself from co-workers (and possibly from recipients as well). Such a person wants to minimize contact with all people and does not want to be bothered by anyone. "Just leave me alone and let me do my job by myself" is the message that comes from the individual who sits off in a corner, does not socialize with co-workers at lunch or coffee breaks, and leaves immediately when the day is done. This self-isolation may develop as a response to the emotional stress of the job—indeed, it is often an important indicator of burnout. Sometimes it occurs in conjunction with "petty bureaucrat," go-strictly-by-the-book behavior. Although such withdrawal may represent an attempt to reduce the amount of interpersonal stress, it has the unintended side effect of reducing the potential for help and support that a worker can receive from his or her fellows.

Isolation from one's peers is not always a deliberate choice. Some helpers may have jobs that keep them at a distance from professional colleagues. For example, isolation can be a hidden cost for providers who solo in private practice. The psychologist who is the sole provider of mental health services in a remote rural area ("out in the boondocks") is effectively cut off from peers who could provide needed support. Teachers who work alone in their own classrooms may also feel isolated, especially if there is little opportunity to get together with fellow teachers down the hall.

The physical arrangement of some job settings can effectively isolate co-workers. Sometimes it is by oversight in the design of the work space, but it may also be a planned way to minimize fraternization.

> The prison guards at one of California's largest state prisons do not even have a locker room where they can change into and out of their uniforms and, while doing so, have a chance to chat with their fellow officers. Says Ben T., "We change in our cars if we don't want our neighbors to know we're prison guards. But it makes you feel real shabby. We don't have time to wind down at the end of our shift by exchanging stories or jokes or whatever with the other guys coming in or leaving with us, as we would if we changed clothes there and had a cup of coffee or something." When a guard does something that puts him in bad with other staff, he finds himself isolated in a gun tower for his entire shift, maybe for weeks on end.

Within many service institutions providers have separate, individual case loads rather than shared ones. To some extent they are in "private practice" even though they work in the same job setting. When there are no shared responsibilities or teamwork or some sort of "buddy system," there are additional emotional pressures on each individual helper. He or she has full responsibility for the recipient, but has less access to peer support—partly because co-workers will be less familiar with the recipient's case, and partly because a request for aid will be viewed as a personal failure ("If I had handled it right, I wouldn't need anybody's help"). Note how the structure of the job setting can create a problem for the provider who, however, interprets it in personal terms—an example of the personalistic bias discussed in Chapter 1. The emotional strain of this kind of job situation is illustrated vividly by the case of Jack C., a child protective services worker in the Southwest.

> In the agency where Jack C. worked, each staff member worked individually with the families on his or her case load. Jack had one family consisting of a woman, her young child, and her common-law husband. There was a great deal of fighting within the family and, over time, increasingly clear signs of child abuse. Although workers are loath actually to remove a child from the family, Jack finally decided that, in this case, all other alternatives had been exhausted and it was the only way to ensure the child's safety. After making arrangements for the removal of the child to a foster family, Jack was suddenly confronted at his desk by the distraught mother, who was brandishing a knife and threatening to kill him. She blamed him personally for the loss of her child and for her feelings of powerlessness and humiliation, and she demanded that he be forbidden to

deal further with her and her family. Clearly, the situation was going from bad to worse, and Jack's supervisor decided to remove him from the case and have another "neutral" worker take over with the family. However, no other worker was as familiar with the case as Jack was, and so it took time and a duplication of some earlier efforts to begin dealing with the family's problems again. Furthermore, Jack viewed his removal from the case as a public sign that he had failed—even though he believed (and everyone assured him) that he had done the right thing. He felt angry at the client for causing the problem, angry at his supervisor for having to make him appear as a failure, and angry at his co-workers—for being witnesses to his "disgrace," for being sympathetic, for *not* having "failed" themselves. Although Jack knew it was better that he not continue with the case, the way the situation had to be handled within the agency left him emotionally exhausted and upset with everyone around him.

SUPERVISORS: HELP OR HINDRANCE?

Just as peer relations can be a source of emotional stress and subsequent burnout, so can relations with one's supervisor. Like a co-worker, a supervisor is yet another human being the helper must deal with constantly—and if the dealings are unsatisfactory the resulting tension and friction add their toll to the emotional overload of the job. Unlike a co-worker, however, a supervisor occupies a position of authority over the helper and has the power to shape and influence the nature of the helper's relationships to recipients. Burnout among providers can be hastened or alleviated by supervisory actions.

Just as helpers and recipients may expect different things from the helping relationship—a mismatch of expectations that can create mutual misunderstanding and animosity—so can helpers and supervisors. They might have different ideas about how to evaluate the helper's work and determine that he or she has done a good job. Frequently, supervisors base their judgments on quantitative dimensions that can be tabulated easily—for example, the number of clients the helper has worked with each day or the number of "successful terminations" per month. However, many providers feel that the quality of their care or service is what should be evaluated. "I can do a good job with twenty-five clients or a mediocre job with twenty-five clients—so the number of people I see doesn't really tell you if I'm providing good service." From the provider's point of view the supervisor is using unimportant or irrelevant criteria to judge performance. But those are the criteria that count, in terms of pay and promotion, and so the provider is pushed to meet the quota. To do so the provider may develop the impersonal "processing" of people that is associated with burnout and that creates client complaints.

The problem is not that supervisors aren't interested in quality of service—they are. But they themselves are under pressure to meet quantitative standards.

The number of people who utilize the services of an institution is often the index of whether its existence is justified. Therefore, administrators will ask supervisors to demonstrate that their employees are, in fact, dealing with sufficiently large numbers of people. Another aspect of this problem is that quality of service is a lot more difficult to measure than quantity. How does a supervisor determine that a helper is conducting "good" interviews? Or providing "appropriate" services? Or being truly "helpful"? The measures that are commonly used still translate into quantity (such as the number of fan letters or complaints). Furthermore, any two people (such as a helper and a supervisor) may disagree on what is actually good or useful to do. For example, a social worker may believe that an extended interview with a client is the best way to establish rapport and understand the client's problems. The supervisor may believe that the extra time is an unnecessary waste since it does not lead to any appreciable change in the worker's final decision.

When helpers and supervisors are at odds over the evaluation of the help given, there is likely to be animosity between them. The helpers will feel dissatisfied with their jobs and may not do more than the bare minimum required. "Why should I knock myself out if it's not going to count for anything? They don't recognize it when I really do my best work, so why bother?" These feelings of dissatisfaction are deepened when helpers fail to get good, clear feedback from their supervisors. Like anyone else, professional providers need to know when they are doing a good job and when they are not. This is especially true when they are responsible for major decisions and may be feeling insecure about the ones they have made. To some extent they can judge their effectiveness for themselves by the outcome of their aid to the recipient. The legal services attorney knows if the client's case was won or lost, the nurse knows if the patient recovered from an illness, and a teacher knows if the student has learned some new material. However, when the outcome is ambiguous or uncertain, this potential source of feedback is lost. For example, did the counseling *really* help the client feel better or make better decisions? The answer may not be clear. Similarly, how can you demonstrate that the service you rendered *prevented* someone from doing something harmful? There is nothing to show for it except the absence of a bad consequence.

Although outcome is important, it is not the only critical aspect of the helping relationship. The *process* by which the outcome is attained may be just as significant (if not more so). Two physicians might prescribe the identical medication for a patient, but one might be more successful than the other in getting the patient to take the medication, return for a follow-up visit, change dietary habits, and so on—largely because of a better "bedside manner" in working with patients.

Evaluation of the process is not self-evident; often it relies on the feedback provided by other people—recipients, co-workers, and supervisors. Feedback from supervisors is especially important for two reasons: it tells providers how well they are doing on the job (and how they might improve), and it lets them know that their work is appreciated and valued. Too often, however, this feedback is not given well. Sometimes it is so vague that it fails to convey much useful information. For example, suppose your supervisor said, "You're doing OK." Does that mean you're doing a good job or an adequate one? What aspects of your work are OK–all or some of them? What do you do that is fine the way it is, and what could be improved? Maybe the vagueness means the supervisor really didn't notice your work, but just needed something to say.

At other times supervisors make more clear, precise, and specific comments. But more often than not, they refer to things the helper did wrong rather than what he or she did right. Negative feedback predominates, while positive feedback is minimal or nonexistent. This is the same pattern of feedback that the helper often gets from recipients. Criticisms and negative comments can be useful, particularly if they are phrased in constructive ways that show the helper how to improve. But usually they are not constructive advice about future ways to behave differently, but are instead blame for past blunders. Being told that you are a "dummy," in so many words, can only make you feel deflated and depressed rather than inspired to try harder.

Even when supervisors have positive things to say to the helper, they often tack on a critical comment as well, and this can undercut the impact of the initial praise. Sometimes this is done to appear more discriminating. A similar approach is taken in popular magazine stories about celebrities, where a little "cut" is thrown in at the end to prevent the essay from being a "puff piece." Diane P., a social worker on the East Coast, described how she feels when a "puff piece" is pricked by the critical "but" that undoes any compliment:

> There never seems to be a time when I hear that I'm doing a good job, period. It's always, "Diane, you're doing a good job, you really are, *but. . . .*" Always "but" and some sort of minor, picky criticism. I've come to distrust the part about doing a good job because I figure it's just a sugar coating to make the criticisms easier to swallow.

Purely positive feedback may not be given as regularly by supervisors because they take it for granted that their employees will provide good service or care–it is only necessary for them to point out when the service falls short. But as we saw in Chapter 2, the pitfall of this approach is that it creates an exclusively negative working environment for the professional helper. With time, this continual gloomy atmosphere can blot out the warmth of care and concern for others, as helpers give out what they get.

Relations with supervisors are also strained if there is little faith or trust. Some providers feel that management is not really behind them, and that if there is any complaint raised by the public, the supervisors will automatically assume that the providers were in the wrong instead of standing up for them. Also, if providers believe that any sign of shortcomings will be used against them, they will be reluctant to let their supervisor know that they have a problem and want some guidance or advice. Helpers can need help too, but if they are unable to get it from their supervisors, they have lost a potential source of support against the onset of burnout. Consider the experience of Marjorie W., a service representative in a Social Security office in the Southeast:

> My burnout was due to too many pressures—from the public who wanted assistance and from management who offered no relief. I was the only service representative in a small office, and I was expected to "do it all." It was not unusual to interview twenty to thirty-five people a day, answer most of the incoming telephone calls and mail, and handle requests for assistance from our program service centers. Most of these contacts represented complaints: "I did not get my check." "How do you expect me to live on this?" "The amount of the check is not correct." "Why can't I work and still get my checks?" In addition to this, our claims staff consisted of inexperienced trainees. Often by the time an individual contacted me for assistance, he (or she) felt he had been given the runaround by inept interviewers and was belligerent at the outset.
>
> I do not feel that management had any sympathy for my plight. I did express how I felt, but the usual response was a shrug and "Well, what's to be done?" After I was threatened by an individual for something I had no hand in and was not responsible for, and in the same week was cussed out over the phone, I decided it was not worth it and requested a lateral reassignment to a noninterviewing position. Management responded by saying *I* could have been the reason these individuals were irate and that there were no noninterviewing positions available. However, I was *not* a goof-off, I was a qualified and competent employee who had received several awards for superior performance.

PLANS, POLICIES, AND PROCEDURES

The nature of the service institution—its goals, its resources, its operating policy—defines and constrains the contact that providers have with recipients. It determines what services will or will not be provided, what people are eligible for them, and what procedures must be followed in the delivery of these services. The institution's impact on the form and content of the helping relationship means that it can play an important role in promoting or alleviating burnout.

Every service institution has its own concept of "successful service." Whether it be to cure illness, or help people in distress, or provide information, or teach new skills, or whatever—the institution is mobilized to achieve that abstract goal. The professional helpers within an institution are also oriented toward that goal, but sometimes they may clash with the institution's management over how best to reach it. When this happens management and employees are fighting each other rather than working together toward their stated objective.

> For example, the mandate for many rehabilitation counselors is to "rehabilitate" their clients—to help them get medical and psychological services, financial aid, a job, and so forth. But, in fact, the counselors disagree with their superiors about what really constitutes successful "rehabilitation." Is it when the client gets a job? When the client has held a job for at least a year? When the client has resolved his psychological hang-ups? Or what? The administration tends to take the short-term estimates, while the counselors take the long-term ones. The administration thinks the counselors spend too much time with each client and therefore see too few of them; the counselors think they have to spend too little time with each client and are therefore unable to help clients get truly rehabilitated. The administration wants to see more clients treated and more completed "successful termination" forms; the counselors feel the number of "terminations" is meaningless, because they don't think they were actually "successful." This recurrent clash of goals places an extra emotional burden on the rehabilitation counselors, since they are caught between the competing demands of their clients and of their superiors. Any effort they put into helping their clients will never be enough, since it will always fall short of success as they have defined it.

Burnout is also affected by institutional rules that structure the nature of the contact between helper and recipient. These rules can introduce new sources of emotional stress or fuel those that are already present. They may require the staff person to do unpleasant tasks (as we saw earlier in the case of the woman collecting payments for hospital bills). They may require that certain questions be asked of recipients—questions that are bound to be embarrassing or upsetting for both people. For example, a social or legal service agency first has to establish a potential client's eligibility for services. This means that the intake interviewer must ask a series of questions about the client's financial status before asking about the client's problems. The client is likely to feel uncomfortable or angry about answering these questions, and the questioner may feel awkward about insisting on the answers.

> Recently, women in Alaska who applied for Aid to Dependent Children had to fill out a form that was designed to establish paternity for children out of wedlock (a necessary requirement for the state to obtain federal funds). The form included the following questions:
>
> - Were you living with the child's father during the ten-month period prior to birth? Where?
> - Number of times you had sex at the above address(es)? Number of times you had sex with the father in the ten months before birth?
> - During which incident do you believe the child was conceived? (Give date and place)

- Did you have sex with any other person during this ten-month period? If so for each person state: (a) Name and address. (b) Dates on which intercourse occurred. (c) Addresses and description of place at which the intercourse occurred.
- Do you have any other children out of wedlock? Are you now keeping company with anyone with whom you are having sexual relations?[11]

In addition to rules that explicitly direct the provider to act in certain ways toward the recipient, the institution may also have rules that limit or forbid certain staff behaviors. For example, the provider may be restricted from providing certain services or granting certain funds. He or she may then be trapped in the uncomfortable position of having to turn people away for reasons that are not always convincing. One welfare worker described her feeling about having to deny additional financial aid to clients: "I just have to tell them to make do. And it hurts. Because I know they can't make do."

Institutional regulations may place time limits on the helper's contact with clients or patients. For instance, psychologists at one university student health center may have no more than four therapy sessions with any one student (for long-term treatment, the student must make arrangements elsewhere). Time constraints are more frequent when the institution must deal with large numbers of people or has limited resources with which to care for them. If the time limits are too restrictive, the helper will have less chance to provide complete and adequate service. Time pressures will also promote impersonal "processing" of recipients.

Many institutions require their staff to take recipients on a "first come, first served" basis. This means that the helpers have no choice of which people to work with and little or no possibility of referring difficult or unpleasant clients to someone else who might work more effectively with them. In one "hotline" suicide prevention center, the rule for staff is, "You pick up the phone, it's *your* call." A staff person who has had several frustrating experiences with a "chronic" caller may get to the point of not wanting to answer the telephone unless he or she knows whether the "chronic" is on the other end of the line. But that cannot be known–to find out who is there, the staff member must pick up the telephone, and at that point he or she has total responsibility for the call. Over time the staff person comes to dread contact with clients. In this sort of situation helpers experience a lack of control over their work and end up feeling "trapped."

A sense of being trapped also occurs when institutional rules require helpers to meet with unwilling recipients. For example, prison psychologists must deal with prisoners who are attending therapy sessions only because they have to in order to be paroled, rather than because they want to. Not only are the prisoners uncooperative and uninterested in the mandatory sessions, but it is unlikely that the therapy, perceived as coercive, will be at all useful or effective. Police must often work with people who don't want the police around or who perceive them as the enemy. The cop might be intervening in a domestic dispute, arresting a suspect, or giving someone a ticket. Not only are the people uncooperative, they may be downright antagonistic toward anything the police officer tries to do. In such circumstances the contact between the police and the public is certain to be unpleasant. Repeated experiences like that can instill a negative, cynical view of people in the cop on the beat.

Clearly, institutional rules and regulations can contribute to the emotional stress of the encounter between provider and recipient. They can also be used to *avoid* stress. Helpers can hide behind rules so as not to get personally involved with recipients. For the petty bureaucrat, rules are absolutes—they apply to everyone and there are no exceptions, no unusual cases, no unique situations that need special attention. A rule is a rule is a rule—the helper simply applies a formula rather than developing a personalized solution. Rules can also be used to avoid taking responsibility for unpopular or painful decisions—"I'm sorry, but it's not *my* fault. Nothing personal, you understand, but those are the rules around here. I don't make them, I just follow them." The impersonal approach of the helper-bureaucrat is portrayed by Erich Fromm in *The Sane Society*:

> The bureaucrat's relationship to people is one of complete alienation. They, the people to be administered, are objects whom the bureaucrats consider . . . completely impersonally; the manager-bureaucrat must not feel, as far as his professional activity is concerned; he must manipulate people as though they were figures or things.[12]

Professional helpers who operate by the rules of the institution are often successful at meeting the goals established by the bureaucracy. However, these goals may conflict with those of the helper's profession, putting the helper in a real bind. The situation facing the rehabilitation counselors mentioned a few pages back illustrates this problem: what was considered successful treatment or rehabilitation of the client by professional standards was too lengthy and costly from the point of view of the bureaucracy. This problem can be exacerbated when there are several different professional groups within one agency (such as social workers, psychologists, and psychiatrists within a community mental health center). Helpers' allegiance to their professions' goals and standards has many benefits, but it also has the potential drawback of disrupting cooperative work within the institution.

In their struggle to provide good service, treatment, or care, providers in institutions often run afoul of bureaucratic red tape. The endless paperwork—documenting information, filling out request forms, writing reports, and so forth—can interfere with the provider's direct work with the recipient, since completing necessary paperwork may have a higher priority within the institution. As one social worker put it, "I sometimes think I spend my life filling out forms in quintuplicate—I never really see clients as much as I should. " Moreover, workers often feel no one ever reads their reports—unless the files have eyes. They are just "make-work"—records kept for the sake of keeping records—not *for* anyone, but only against the future possibility of a lawsuit for negligence or malpractice. While paperwork is necessary to requisition funds, equipment, or other resources, it can also be a factor in their slow delivery. A disabled client who needs homemaker services or an elderly client who needs medical treatment might have to wait for days or even weeks to obtain them because of bureaucratic red tape, and that can only arouse frustration and anger on both sides of the helping relationship.

Poor organization and poor management of an organization also contribute to burnout. If the goals of the agency are not clear, if the roles for the staff are ill defined, if bureaucratic hassles predominate, if communication between management and staff is unclear and nonsupportive–then the helper will find it especially difficult to provide good service, treatment, instruction, or care to recipients. A study of child-care agencies found that burnout was highest among staff in agencies that were managed badly.[13] In addition to being poorly organized internally, some institutions may be unclear about their relation to the community. This can lead the community to make improper referrals to the institution or use it as a "dumping ground" for all sorts of problems that the agency is not equipped to handle. For example, a community mental-health center may get saddled with clients who are more appropriately handled by the correctional system, thereby leading to people getting the runaround, lots of wasted time and paperwork that could have been avoided, and bad vibes all around.

Many educational and service institutions have the added burden of receiving little or no support from the public. The community may not approve of the services that are being provided (such as abortions or welfare benefits), or it may be upset or frightened by the agency (such as halfway houses for former convicts or mental patients). There may be a social stigma attached to the job, as many police and prison guards have discovered. When Earl P., a guard at San Quentin, is asked what he does for a living, he gives some vague answer like, "I'm a civil servant" or "I work for the state." In other cases, the community may believe that the institution has failed to do what it was supposed to do. Thus, teachers are often criticized personally for the decline in education and for not having taught Johnny and Jane to read, write, and do adequate arithmetic:

> Dick L., an elementary school teacher, is finding it increasingly uncomfortable to have a drink in the local bar after work. Once some other customers discover he is a teacher, they let him know the contempt they have for his profession–"You guys are doing a lousy job of teaching, and yet you have the nerve to demand bigger salaries. And you already get three months of vacation!" And so on, and so on.

Providing education, service, or treatment is an enormously demanding task in and of itself. But when there is no outside support for this kind of work, then the struggle to serve and the commitment to care may crumble and burn out completely.

BURNOUT[14]

I used to care,
But I don't care much any more.
I used to care
That children had to sit still and be quiet
And read pages 9 to 17
And answer the odd numbered questions at the end of the chapter;
But I don't care much any more.

I used to care
That finishing the assignment is more important than learning the skill,
And getting the right answer is more important than understanding,
And apologizing is more important than being penitent;
But I don't care much any more.

I used to wake up in the night
And think about ways to teach children
To set goals and work toward them,
To make decisions and live with the results,
To work together.
But there were those who felt threatened
And those who felt frightened
Because my classroom was different.
Parents did not understand.
They listened to the evil insinuations and the confidential criticisms.
Their protests overwhelmed my sand-based supports.
I used to care,
But I don't care much any more.

Now I say
Sit down
Be quiet
Read pages 9 to 17
No exciting ideas disturb my sleep.
I haven't had a complaint in over a year.
Nobody seems to care
That I don't care much any more.

Thus, some work contexts can crush the best intentions of a professional provider who brings to the job high ideals and a desire to help others. The central aspect of this work context is the provider-recipient relationship, but it is embedded in layers of other interrelated contexts. There are the provider and co-workers; the provider and supervisors; the supervisors and those to whom they are accountable; the interplay between provider, other staff, and the rules, goals, and status of the institution; and, finally, the context of the institution within the larger community. When most of these contexts are supportive of the provider's role definition and sense of professional worth, he or she can tolerate some disequilibrium in a few. But when many of these contexts are out of sync and not working for the professional provider, the risk of burning out is high.

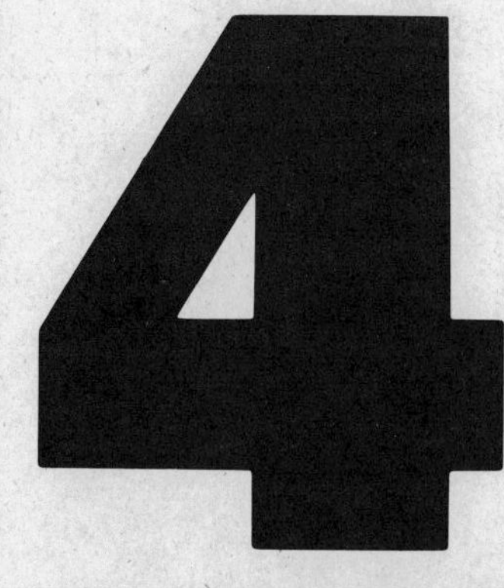

PERSONAL CHARACTERISTICS AS A SOURCE OF BURNOUT

When my marriage went bad I probably started looking for more positives in my job—things that were lacking in the family relationships. I was needing more approval or a feeling of success, accomplishment. When my supervisor would not complete an evaluation after I did an especially good job, I felt bad. It would have meant so much to me.

Ms. K., social worker[1]

Persons entering the helping professions often have high needs for approval and heightened expectations of themselves. Their ability to help others represents, in part, a means to gain social approval and enhance self-image; such individuals receive great satisfaction from the results of their treatment. If work becomes the primary means by which they enhance their self-concept, these persons may overcommit their time and energy. Consequently, they develop few activities, other than work, which produce enjoyment or satisfaction. Eventually, such individuals become burdened by fatigue and are less effective in their primary sphere of gratification, and they receive fewer rewards for their increased labor. The resulting frustration spurs them to more work and begins the vicious cycle which produces burnout. Prior to burnout, these individuals are seen as being

> highly competent and aggressive, and they are respected by both their patients and their colleagues. Their marriages and their relationships with their children begin to suffer, depriving them of their main source of non-work-related support. As marital tensions and interpersonal distances from family increase, they are driven to seek still more work-related satisfaction. Characteristically, they take on more and more responsibility and increase their work schedule, and they seem to seek out situations which result in physical and emotional pressure.[2]

So far, we have seen how burnout is produced by the surrounding situation. The emotional intensity of involvement with people, the negative focus on problems, the lack of positive feedback, or poor peer contact in the job setting are some of the external factors that can elicit burnout. But external factors are not the entire story of burnout; internal factors play an important role as well.

What a person brings to a situation is just as critical as what the situation brings out of (or puts into) him or her. And what a person brings are individual characteristics such as motivations, needs, values, self-esteem, emotional expressiveness and control, and personal style. These internal qualities determine how someone handles external sources of emotional stress and help explain why Person A will experience burnout in a particular work setting while Person B will not. They are also implicated in an individual's original choice of a helping profession as a career.

The relevance of personal characteristics is especially great for people-work professions. Unlike other jobs, where only technical skills are required, these professions call for the use of interpersonal skills as well. The provider must be empathic and understanding, calm and objective while dealing with intimate information, and ready to give help and reassurance. The provider's ability in these areas is largely a function of his or her personality and life experiences. This is especially true if there has been no explicit job training in interpersonal skills. Thus, personality and other personal qualities have a very significant part to play in burnout.

The basic question in this chapter is "*who* is more at risk for burnout?" What demographic traits characterize these people, and do they have a certain type of personality? This *who* question is not putting the blame on someone (as was the *who* question posed in Chapter 1). Rather, it is an attempt to discover just what makes someone more susceptible to burnout and to understand why this should be so.

DEMOGRAPHIC CHARACTERISTICS

The search for who is more vulnerable begins with a look at basic demographic variables. Are there differences in burnout as a function of sex, ethnic background, age, marital and family status, and education? To answer these questions, Susan Jackson and I have had the Maslach Burnout Inventory (MBI) completed by a wide range of human services professionals from various parts of the United States.[3] The results of this survey reveal interesting patterns of burnout, and I will speculate on some of their underlying reasons.

Sex

Overall, men and women are fairly similar in their experience of burnout. This basic similarity should be kept in mind when considering the differences, which are rather small. Essentially, these differences are that men show slightly more of one aspect of burnout, and women show slightly more of another. Women tend to experience more emotional exhaustion, and to experience it more intensely, than men. However, men are more likely to have depersonalized and callous feelings about the people they work with. This variation may reflect differences in masculine and feminine sex roles. Women are expected to be more oriented toward people than are men—they are supposed to be nurturant, sociable, and sensitive to people's feelings. They are also supposed to be very emotional people themselves, while men are supposed to be hard, tough, and unemotional (the "big boys don't cry" stereotype). Because of these differences in the way men and women are brought up, they may have different strengths and weaknesses with respect to burnout. To the extent that women are more likely to get emotionally involved with people, they run a greater risk of emotional exhaustion. To the extent that men are less oriented toward close contact with people, they are more prone to exhibit depersonalization.

It is also possible, however, that these sex differences in burnout reflect the different occupations that men and women have, rather than differences in masculine and feminine traits. Many people-work jobs are sex segregated—they are either done mostly by men or mostly by women (rather than by both sexes equally). For example, most physicians, police officers, and psychiatrists are men, while most nurses, social workers, and counselors are women. Thus, the different patterns of burnout displayed by male physicians and female nurses may actually reflect differences in their contact with patients, their power and status within the hospital, and so forth. However, my research has found that the differences between "women's work" and "men's work" are not the whole story. There is still something about the personal qualities that distinguish the two sexes that makes depersonalization more of a problem for men, and emotional exhaustion more of a problem for women.

Ethnic Background

The vast majority of the people workers I have studied have been Caucasian. This is not surprising, given that whites are the majority group in the United States, but it also reflects the underrepresentation of ethnic minorities in some helping professions. The fact that our information about minorities and burnout is based on a much smaller group of people means that we have to be cautious about conclusions drawn from the comparisons.

Burnout, as I have described it thus far, can be considered the white experience of this phenomenon. It can also be used as the standard against which to compare the experiences of ethnic minorities. The question is whether there are any noteworthy differences for these minority groups. In the case of Asian-American helpers, the answer is "no." Burnout among Asian-American helpers is very similar to that of whites. This similarity far outweighs the slight differences that have been found, but these differences are consistently in the direction of more burnout for Asian Americans. They report slightly more emotional exhaustion, slightly more depersonalization, and a somewhat lower sense of accomplishment in their work with people.

In contrast, there are dramatic differences in burnout between black and white helping professionals. Compared to whites, blacks do not burn out as much. They experience much less emotional exhaustion and much less depersonalization. This is true for both the frequency and the intensity of these feelings. Why should blacks function better in the same jobs that lead whites to burn out? One possibility is that they come from communities in which there is a greater emphasis on family and friendship networks and on direct, one-on-one relationships with people. "Rapping" with each other involves emotional expression, confrontation, personal feedback, and resolutions of conflicts; there is also more assertiveness and spontaneity. Consequently, blacks may be more experienced in dealing directly with people, even in emotionally charged situations, than are whites. Furthermore, they may be more prepared to deal with problems and pain, since it is likely that they have experienced them more in their own lives (because of discrimination and poverty) than whites have. The troubles they have already seen may give them a more balanced and realistic perspective on the ones yet to come for them and those they work with. Knowing already that the world cannot be changed overnight, they will be less disillusioned the next morning when it has not.

So far in my research the number of other ethnic minorities (Latinos, Native Americans, and so on) has been too small to be a basis for separate group comparisons—a weakness that will be rectified in future studies. However, when combined into a single group, they show a pattern that is closer to the black experience than to the white. That is, they report less emotional exhaustion and less depersonalization (although, like Asian Americans, they also experience less personal accomplishment).

Age

There is a clear relationship between age and burnout. Burnout is greatest when people workers are young and is lower for older workers. Younger people usually have less work experience than older ones, but it turns out that the effect of age reflects more than just the length of time on the job. "Older but wiser" seems to be the case here—with increased age, people are more stable and mature, have a more balanced perspective on life, and are less prone to the excesses of burnout.

There is another reason for the relationship of burnout to youth. In many of my research interviews people said that the first bout with burnout was likely to happen in the first few years of one's career. The period of time most often cited in one psychiatric ward was one and a half years, poverty lawyers spoke of a reduction of the former four-year stint to two, and for many social services agencies the critical period for burnout was between one and five years on the job. If people have difficulty in dealing with burnout at this point, when they are younger and newer to the job, they may leave the profession entirely. Because of this early dropout of the burned out, they will not be around five or ten years later to answer questions about the emotional strain of their work. In other words, the older people workers are the survivors—the ones who managed to handle the early threat of burnout and stayed on to do well in their careers. Not surprisingly, then, they report less burnout than their younger colleagues.

Marital and Family Status

Burnout also has a consistent relationship with marital status. People workers who are single experience the most burnout, while those who are married experience the least. Providers who are divorced generally fall in between these two groups; they are closer to the singles in terms of higher emotional exhaustion, but closer to the marrieds in terms of lower depersonalization and greater sense of accomplishment.

Just as being unmarried is associated with a greater risk of burnout, so is being childless. Contrary to the view that children are an additional emotional burden (which should exacerbate burnout), burnout is less for professional helpers with families.

> My colleagues and I investigated the relation between burnout and family life in a nationwide study of public contact employees in the Social Security Administration. While married employees showed less burnout than singles, we found an even more striking difference between those who had children and those who did not. Compared to employees who had one or more children, childless employees reported much more emotional exhaustion and depersonalization, and a much lower sense of personal accomplishment. Moreover, childless employees expressed a far greater desire to spend *less* time working with the public.[4]

There are several reasons why people with families are less vulnerable to burnout. First, they tend to be older, more stable, and psychologically mature individuals. Second, their involvement with a spouse and children makes them more experienced in dealing with personal problems and emotional conflicts. Third, a family is often an emotional resource, rather than an emotional drain (as we shall see in Chapters 6 and 7). The love and support of family members help the individual cope with the emotional demands of work. Finally, the person with a family has a different view of the job than does the person who is single. Having a family to support makes the practitioner more realistically concerned about job security, salary, and benefits (and maybe less idealistic), as compared to the childless employee, who feels more free to move and change jobs than to toler ate difficult ones. Furthermore, the family man or woman does not depend so heavily on the job as a source of his or her personal social life. Since the family fulfills many of the person's needs for affection and approval, there is less reason to seek personal gratification from clients or colleagues (and thus to get emotionally entangled with them).

Education

Professional helpers are a highly educated group, since the majority of them have gone to college, and many have had postgraduate training. People with different amounts of education are not dramatically different with respect to burnout–as with the variable of sex, the similarities are more striking than the differences. However, the differences we did find are fairly consistent, but complex.

In general, the greatest amount of burnout is found for providers who have completed college but have not had any postgraduate training. They show the most depersonalization and the least personal accomplishment, and they tend to have more emotional exhaustion. Interestingly, we also found a high degree of emotional exhaustion for providers with postgraduate training–although on all other dimensions of burnout this group scores the lowest. Overall, we found less burnout for providers with less education, and in particular for those who have had some college experience but not a full four years.

What do these results mean? One possible explanation is that people with different amounts of education enter different types of jobs. The person who never completed college will not become a physician, for example. Thus, the differences between these groups reflect, in large part, the emotional demands of the work these people perform and not simply their educational background. Education and occupation are interrelated. This may be the reason why the most highly trained helpers experience emotional exhaustion but not the other aspects of burnout. The nature of their jobs may cause greater emotional stress, but their training has equipped them to cope more successfully with it.

People with higher levels of education have higher expectations for what they want to do in life. They may be very idealistic and aspire to great things. However, if they are not prepared well for the reality of their helper role, the clash of this reality with their ideals can result in disillusionment and burnout. Helpers who have had less schooling may not have such high aspirations, and so there is less of a gap between their goals and their actual achievements. If a person's education provides noble goals and the inspiration to achieve them, but neglects to provide practical training, then that person is being set up for a bad case of burnout. This could explain why college-educated helpers are more vulnerable to burnout than those with additional postgraduate studies. This further training is usually oriented toward pragmatic skills as well as being a ticket to better jobs.

PERSONALITY

Burnout does not occur for all of the people all of the time. There are clearly individual variations in the overall pattern—variations that seem to be related to differences in individual personality. By *personality* I mean the essential character of an individual—the mental, emotional, and social qualities or traits that combine into a unique whole. One's interpersonal style, method of handling problems, expression and control of emotions, and conception of self are all aspects of personality that have special significance for burnout.

Having noted that there are individual differences in vulnerability to burnout, some people are content to let it go at that. "You know that there are going to be some people who can't handle things and will burn out, and that there are others who will breeze through it all—that's just the way people are." However, attributing burnout to individual idiosyncrasies provides little insight. We need to go beyond the fact that certain people do burn out and discover just what kind of people they are.

Bound for Burnout: A Personality Profile

The first clues about the personal roots of burnout come from recent studies done by two of my doctoral students, Maxine Gann and Steve Heckman.[5] A portrait of the provider who is almost predestined for problems emerges from these research results.

The burnout-prone individual is, first of all, someone who is weak and unassertive in dealing with people. Such a person is submissive, anxious, and fearful of involvement and has difficulty in setting limits within the helping relationship. This person is often unable to exert control over a situation and will passively yield to its demands rather than actively limiting them to his or her capacity to give. It is easy for this person to become overburdened emotionally, and so the risk of emotional exhaustion is high.

The burnout-prone individual is also someone who is impatient and intolerant. Such a person will get easily angered and frustrated by any obstacles in his or her path and may have difficulty controlling any hostile impulses. He or she is likely to project these feelings onto clients and to treat them in more depersonalized and derogatory ways.

Finally, the burnout-prone individual is someone who lacks self-confidence, has little ambition, and is more reserved and conventional. Such a person has neither a clearly defined set of goals nor the determination and self-assurance needed to achieve them. He or she acquiesces and adapts to the constraints of the situation, rather than confronting the challenges and being more forceful and enterprising. Faced with self-doubts this person tries to establish a sense of self-worth by winning the approval and acceptance of other people. In so doing the person may be so accommodating that he or she is overextended too often. This individual is more easily discouraged by difficulties and does not feel a sense of personal accomplishment and effectiveness in dealing with people.

This character sketch of the high-risk burnout personality is a composite of several key characteristics. It would be a mistake to assume that people who match this composite are the *only* ones at risk for burnout. Everyone is at risk, to some extent, if the emotional stress of the work becomes excessive, but those with a certain personal makeup will be even more so at any given level of work stress. Furthermore, we should not assume that *all* of these characteristics have to be present before considering the person at risk—any one of them can make a person more vulnerable to some aspect of burnout. Thus, we need to consider each of these characteristics separately to get a more complete understanding of how they are linked to the burnout syndrome.

Self-Concept

Your own sense of who you are, and your evaluation of that unique being, play an important role in your relations with the people around you. To know thyself and like thyself is critical for giving of thyself unto others.

ESTEEM AND CONFIDENCE If you look at the person you are and are *not* pleased and impressed with what you see—"I'm not so great," "I can never do anything right," "nobody really likes me," "I haven't got much to show for my life"—then you are going to have trouble with burnout. The demands of a helping relationship can be difficult under any circumstances, but they can be overwhelming if you have little faith that you can meet its challenges.

For one thing, you are less strong and assertive in your dealings with people if you lack confidence in yourself. You defer and acquiesce, instead of determine and initiate. You have a passive and powerless position instead of an active and autonomous one. You are at the mercy of the surrounding situation, instead of shaping and controlling it. As a result you have a greater chance of being overburdened and emotionally depleted by the helping situations in which you work.

Obstacles loom much larger when you suffer from low self-esteem. Any kind of setback or snafu becomes a major crisis, even an insurmountable one, in your eyes. You are less willing to push ahead and try to overcome these obstacles ("Why bother? I know I can't do it anyway") and more willing to give up when things get tough ("See? I told you I couldn't do it"). This lack of drive and determination makes the cycle self-perpetuating–if you fold in the face of frustrations, this will only confirm your poor judgment of yourself, which will, in turn, give you even more reason not to try harder.

A poor self-concept is self-perpetuating in another way as well. It leads you to focus selectively on your failures rather than your successes. When you think badly about yourself, all the evidence that supports that conclusion is most salient in your mind. That is, you remember more of the things that went wrong than those that went right. You carry this negative frame of reference with you into each new situation, and it affects what you learn from these experiences.

> An analogy can be made here to the classic difference between the optimist and the pessimist. Upon seeing a bowl of water in which the water is at the halfway mark, the optimist will say it is half-full while the pessimist will say it is half-empty. In a similar way, the provider with high self-esteem and the one with low self-esteem will see the exact same helping situation very differently and will learn very different things from it. The high self-esteem person will focus more on what went well, while the low self-esteem person will focus more on what went poorly. Even if the situation turns out to be a disaster, the positive, "half-full" orientation of the high self-esteem provider will still triumph–"What can I learn from all this, so that I can do better next time?" No matter what the setbacks, they are unlikely to shake the foundation of a solid faith in oneself.

If you lack a sense of self-worth, you do not have the basic assurance that you are a good person who is doing some good things. Instead, you are likely to be seeking this assurance from others. One of the reasons you might have chosen to be in a helping profession is to use it to alleviate any sense of worthlessness–"I can't be all bad if I do some good." The drawback of being so dependent on others for this type of self-validation is that you are likely to be emotionally devastated if people fail to provide it. And, as we have seen, factors in the helping professions operate against getting positive feedback. Thus, by constantly relying on others as a test of your self-worth ("Am I OK?" "Is this good enough?"), you make yourself more vulnerable to burnout when they either don't answer or say "no."

LIMITS AND RESPONSIBILITIES It is not only how you feel about yourself that is important for burnout, but how well you know and understand the human being you are. What are your skills and talents–and what are your deficiencies? What are your strong points–and what are your weak spots? What is the range of your capabilities–and what are their limits?

If you do not know the answers to these questions and are insensitive to your minuses (as well as to your pluses), you will be more vulnerable to burnout. Why? Because ignorance of your limits means you are likely to exceed them. The emotional overload that precipitates burnout is more likely to occur if you do not know when it is time to stop, to say no, or to make changes.

The failure to recognize personal limits is especially critical in helping professions, where people are dealing with other people's lives. All too often providers feel completely responsible for whether a client succeeds or fails, lives or dies—and are emotionally overwhelmed by this heavy burden. This unwarranted sense of responsibility is usually tied to feelings of omnipotence—feelings that "I know it all and I can do it all." When these fantasies of omnipotence are not tempered by the recognition of actual limitations, ideals and expectations will be out of touch with reality. As a result, there will be discrepancies between aspirations and actual achievements—and feelings of failure will be sure to follow.

Personal Needs

All of us have basic psychological needs that we strive to fulfill. We want to be loved and cherished, admired and respected by other people. We also want to *be* somebody—to make our mark in the world, achieve success, and be recognized and praised for these accomplishments. Although these needs are common to everyone, they vary in importance for different individuals. The strength of these needs, and the way they are (or are not) satisfied, have important implications for burnout.

APPROVAL AND AFFECTION The need to be liked and approved of by other people is clearly a critical personality factor in burnout. When this need is strong the provider will be very dependent on the whims and wishes of clients and colleagues and will work hard to please them and to satisfy their demands. He or she will not do anything that might upset people (such as saying no or disagreeing with them), since that might cause them to withdraw their approval. Should appreciation not be forthcoming from these people, the provider will feel hurt and betrayed and will begin to dislike and disparage them.

The need to be liked by the people at work will become excessive when there are few other sources of affection in the provider's life. The person who lacks close relationships with friends or family will be far more dependent on clients and colleagues for signs of appreciation.

> An example is the social worker quoted at the beginning of this chapter—when she was no longer getting approval at home, she looked even harder for it at the office. Or think back to Betty G., the teacher in Chapter 1, who said that she had no one to come home to except the cat. The most important people in her life were her students, and she knocked herself out trying to please them and be loved by them.

ACHIEVEMENT The need to achieve is what spurs all of us on to do more and better things, despite the obstacles in our path. It is a critical personality factor in the success of many helping professionals, who must undertake years of hard work in preparation for their eventual careers. However, problems arise when the need to achieve becomes so strong that all else is sacrificed to satisfying it. The detrimental effects of overachievement are illustrated by the experience of some physicians:

> Obligatory achievement is one manifestation of the obsessive character more likely to occur in those reared by autocratic and restrictive parents. Overachievement emerges when the child feels that he can maintain self-esteem only by satisfying the demands of others. Inherent in the socialization of physicians are factors that reinforce this overachievement; in some cases, these factors help produce doctors who can maintain self-esteem only through compulsive self-denial. These physicians have particular difficulty satisfying their demands for nurturance and typically will experience guilt whenever they receive help from others. Some solace can be achieved by satisfying the demands of patients; identification with the dependent patient may vicariously satisfy nurturance needs of these physicians. Unaccustomed to appreciating personal needs, the physician can saturate his life with professional obligations while at the same time leaving little opportunity for the cultivation of recreational skills or relationships with friends or with family. Ultimately, frank depression emerges.[6]

Achievement needs are also related to burnout in another way. When you strive for goals that are vague and unclear ("I just want to make the world a better place") or that are unrealistically high, you are setting yourself up for failure. You will fall short of these great expectations more often than you will meet them, and the losses will outnumber the gains. If this "no-win" experience occurs often, it can have a very detrimental effect on your sense of competence and self-esteem and may lead you to find someone else to blame for the failures. As we shall see in Chapters 6 and 8, there are better ways to establish goals and to achieve them.

AUTONOMY AND CONTROL The need to be independent and self-determining is a hallmark of personal growth and maturity. We want the freedom to choose, and the power to carry out our choices, rather than always being told what to do. People who feel they have some say in their work and can exert control over it are happier with their jobs and with themselves. But if they feel helpless, powerless, and trapped (by the demands of other people or by the restrictions of the job), the betting is that they will burn out.

While burnout is linked to the situational experience of lack of control, it is also tied to the personality factor of an excessive need for control. This need to control everyone and everything, and to refuse to share or delegate power, is characteristic of the authoritarian personality type. According to Herbert

Freudenberger, the authoritarian individual is especially prone to burn out because of this tendency to do it all, to take on too much, and to overextend him- or herself.[7] In addition, authoritarians have a negative, power-based orientation toward people in general, and this can easily feed into the callous cynicism of burnout.

Personal Motivations

What is it that leads people to enter a career of caregiving? Why do they choose to help, cure, teach, nurture as their life's work? For some helping occupations the traditional motivators of good salary, special benefits, and high prestige are almost nonexistent, so personal, intrinsic motives become especially important. Some of these personal motives pose special risks for burnout, so it is critical, both for emotional survival and effectiveness as a helper, that people understand their reasons for giving.

At first glance, caregiving appears to stem from altruistic and selfless motives, in which others and their well-being take precedence over oneself. In our society these motives are held up as noble ideals and are strongly applauded when they appear. But there are other reasons why people help, although they are usually not thought to be quite so noble and praiseworthy—in fact, they are considered somewhat selfish. People may be less willing to acknowledge that these motives are operating even when they are, because they seem inappropriate or unacceptable. Indeed, these motives do raise some potential problems, which I shall discuss later. However, ignoring or denying their existence is not a productive approach; these motives are powerful and need to be openly recognized and understood.

The "selfish" reasons for helping others involve the gratification of personal needs. That is, your involvement with recipients enables you to satisfy some of your own wants and desires. Some helpers have a strong need for approval and affection, which can be satisfied by expressions of appreciation from grateful recipients. Some people may become helpers to gain a sense of self-worth or to give a boost to their self-esteem. Other helpers may be motivated by feelings of guilt, which they hope to expiate through their good deeds. Still others, who may have difficulty in establishing close personal relationships, may use the helping situation as a way of satisfying their need for intimacy.

> The Los Angeles Suicide Prevention Center, like many other such facilities, uses trained volunteers to staff its program and answer incoming calls. What kind of person would seek out this kind of work? A study of these volunteers and their general orientation toward others, came up with an intriguing finding. Although the volunteers were interested in having a close relationship with someone, they themselves did not want to make the first move. Rather, they wanted the other person to initiate the contact and get the interpersonal ball rolling. In other words, they wanted

> intimacy but preferred a passive role in obtaining it. What is interesting here is that the volunteer's job is particularly well suited for satisfying that personal need. The contact with callers is often intimate and intense, since it focuses on major life problems, but the *callers* initiate it. The volunteers do not actively seek out the contacts—they simply wait for the call for help.[8]

In addition to satisfying personal needs, helping relationships may be used as vehicles for personal growth—for the helper, and not just for the recipient.

> In their interviews with me, several psychotherapists mentioned that they had expected to achieve self-actualization through their work, to realize their full potential as human beings, and to discover the real meaning of life. They were disappointed and depressed that enlightenment had not come and were beginning to realize that they were asking too much of the job—that it might provide some, but certainly not all, of the personal gains that they had hoped for.

In some cases, helping people is not viewed as just a job but as an expression of one's personal identity. The individual who takes on the role of rescuer (see Chapter 2) is an example of this; so is the ex-teacher who told me, "Teaching was my ministry, my life." People may also enter certain helping occupations as a way of working out their own problems. For example, several family therapists mentioned their own family difficulties as the factor propelling them into this line of work. Other people may want to avoid dealing with their personal problems and will enter a helping career to focus on someone else's troubles instead of their own.

Self-serving motives are not necessarily bad motives. Achieving satisfaction through one's work and feeling good about oneself are reasonable rewards to expect. However, there are some real dangers in using the helping relationship to obtain personal gratification. Not only can it interfere with the quality of the care that is provided, but it can be a source of great emotional stress and subsequent burnout. Clients cannot provide for the needs of the caregiver (nor should they be expected to). Consequently, the caregiver may be frustrated by not getting all the affection, approval, intimacy, or identity that he or she wants from them. This frustration is likely to be expressed in hostility toward the clients and may be accompanied by depression as well. Psychotherapists have long been aware of the personal pitfalls of countertransference. To avoid them, psychoanalyst Frieda Fromm-Reichmann has argued that the therapist must have a well-developed private life in which personal needs are so well satisfied that the therapist will not be tempted to use the patient relationship for this purpose.[9]

Emotional Control

It should be clear by now that strong emotions are a significant part of helping relationships. Thus the expression and control of these emotions is another personality factor related to the experience of burnout.

HOSTILITY Providing care is often a difficult process, and frustrations and failures are more apt to be common than rare. Feelings of anger and irritation will be relatively frequent. Providers who are unable to deal with these feelings constructively will vent their hostility on other people—usually clients or colleagues (since they are the most easily available targets), but sometimes family or friends as well. There is a search for someone to blame and a desire to get back at them for whatever they did "wrong." An illustration of this type of client-directed hostility is the psychiatrist who views suicide attempts by patients as personal insults to the therapist:

> Dear Ann Landers:
>
> I am a psychiatrist and psychoanalyst who has worked very arduously to humanize the demoralized and sick people who come to me.
>
> I want to comment on the letter from the eighteen-year-old woman who felt cruelly rejected by her therapist. He refused to see her again after she had attempted suicide.
>
> People need to understand that in order to be even marginally successful, therapy must be a two-way street. If I had worked with someone in the extremely demanding and trusting relationship that constitutes psychiatric treatment and that person had tried to punish me by trying to take her life, I would find it very difficult to trust her ever again. What's more, if I were to forgive and try to work with her again, her respect for me and for our work together would be diminished to the point that it would be worthless.
>
> Everyone, patient or not, must accept responsibility for his own behavior. It was extremely useful for that patient to be faced with the fact that one cannot be capricious with the efforts of others and expect the insulted and injured to turn the other cheek. No one, sick or well, should be let off free when he or she indulges in destructive behavior.[10]

In addition to seeking a scapegoat, helpers may express hostility toward others for reasons related to their self-concept. Hostility may serve the hydraulic function of boosting one's self-esteem by putting other people down.

FEAR Some occupations involve serious physical or psychological threats to the helper's well-being, and so the ability to cope with fear is particularly important. For example, police officers and prison guards have to do their job knowing that they might be suddenly attacked, injured, or even killed. Health professionals have to deal with their fear of death and of personal loss, since there is always the chance that their patients will not survive.

All too often, people fail to confront their fears. Either they avoid or deny them, or they try to block off their emotional reactions through a process of "psychic numbing."[11] It may be easier and less immediately painful to flee from fear, but flight does not allow you to come to terms with it. And you *must* come to terms with fear if you want to be effective in your work and maintain your emotional health as well.

> Fear is a common experience for prison guards, but they are often constrained from expressing or even acknowledging it because of an institutional "macho" code that regards emotions as unmasculine. One consequence of this is the channeling of this fear and tension into psychosomatic symptoms, such as neck and back problems, ulcers, and so on. As one former prison guard told me, "Male identity is a killing factor within the all-male prison society. Concern of any kind is all too often translated as weakness. All new correctional officers must learn to control their emotions, especially the incredible fear. Each of us reacted to the fear in our own way—but we had no way to release tensions."

IMPATIENCE Burnout is more of a problem for people with a short fuse. If they are impulsive, impatient, and intolerant, their level of emotional exhaustion is bound to be high, and their feelings about people are likely to become negative.

> Carla L., an attorney in Washington, observed this type of personal trait in her colleagues: "I find the attorneys in legal aid offices much more personable, sensitive, not so pompous—but equally, if not more so, high-strung and short-tempered. And they do move on to other jobs pretty quickly."

A major drawback of this impatient and impulsive style is that you do not give yourself the time to reflect, to gain perspective, and to be more calm, cool, and collected when decisions have to be made. Not only is impatience an emotionally debilitating style, but it may be an ineffective and unproductive way to deal with people's problems, since it increases the risk of making mistakes.

EMPATHY The ability to be empathic—to understand and share in people's experiences—has been regarded as a critical personal trait for many helping professions. The distinction between emotional empathy and cognitive empathy may have important implications for burnout. Understanding someone's problem and seeing things from his or her point of view should enhance your ability to provide good service or care. However, the vicarious experience of that person's emotional turmoil will increase your susceptibility to emotional exhaustion. Emotional empathy is really a sort of weakness or vulnerability, rather than a strength. The person whose feelings are easily aroused (but not necessarily easily controlled) is going to have far more difficulty in dealing with emotionally stressful situations than the person who is less excitable and more psychologically detached. Emotional empathy is akin to wearing your heart on your sleeve—your feelings and concern are up front and very visible, but they are very vulnerable as well. And with repeated bruisings, that heart may get too hard and calloused to feel much any more: "Frankly, client, I don't give a damn."

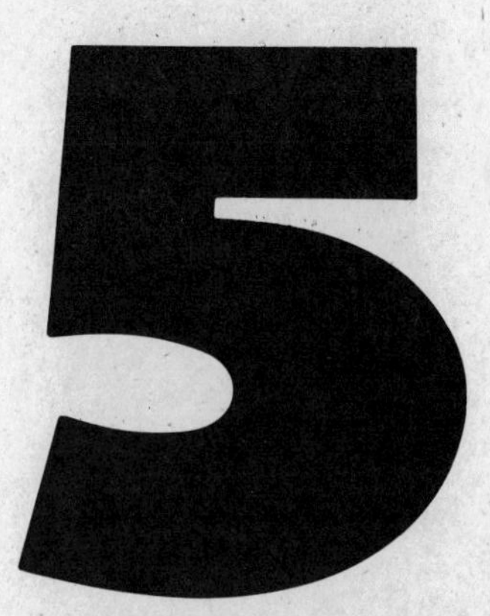

THE EFFECTS OF BURNOUT

I am a social worker in an aging and adult service unit in Florida. I deal in crisis cases concerning alcoholics, mental health problems, and adult abuse, plus regular maintenance cases involving nursing home placements, aftercare follow-up, food stamp evaluation, and general social work. I have reached the point where I simply want to scream for the telephone to stop ringing. I'm even afraid to answer the phone at home and I don't; my wife does and screens the calls, telling the clients or police that I'll return the call. I've been working for fourteen straight months, plus nights and weekends on call duty. I recently received a call at home and had to go out at night, and while I was getting dressed, I was screaming and cursing these motherfuckers for calling me with their goddamned problems, but I didn't even realize it until I returned home and my wife told me I had almost scared our little girl to death. She's four years old, and she wanted to know why Daddy was so mad and upset, and I honestly didn't even know I had lost control of myself. Really I didn't.

Robert T., social worker

James is a New York cop who joined the force in 1966. His first assignment involved "fixers"—checking an abandoned building or guarding the

> home of a dignitary. "It didn't matter whether I showed up for work or not," he says, and soon he began to have a few drinks with the guys instead. He was later assigned to a public-morals squad. Although he disliked having to hassle prostitutes, he found the job exciting. "But I did have to go into movie houses and pick up homosexuals in the act. Whenever I had to do a job like that I had a couple of drinks. . ." In 1971, two policemen were killed in an ambush. "I had known them. . . . the way they got killed landed me in a period of deep depression. There's no justice. They were nice guys. My release for that was a drink." James found it difficult to get up in the mornings to go to work, his memory became faulty, and he failed to keep good records for court testimony. To unwind after work, he would have several drinks. In 1972, while checking out a narcotics drop, James was almost killed. Although he felt he had done a heroic act, the department did not share that view and removed him from plainclothes duty—which ruined his chances of ever becoming a detective. While drinking in a Brooklyn bar, James got into an argument with another man. After grappling with him, James told him he was under arrest and then fired his gun. Luckily, the man's belt buckle deflected the bullet and so his injury was not fatal.[1]

People pay a heavy price for being their brother's (and sister's) keeper. The emotional exhaustion and cynicism of burnout are often accompanied by a deterioration in physical and psychological well-being. Relationships with other people suffer, both on and off the job. These negative side effects are not unique to burnout—indeed, they are common correlates of other forms of stress. But the fact that they do flare up when burnout occurs suggests that the syndrome is a far more serious problem than we had previously thought. The burned-out provider is prone to health problems, psychological impairment, loss of self-esteem, and a growing dissatisfaction with the job. However, the damaging impact of burnout goes beyond the individual caregiver. It can hurt the recipients, who receive less good service and are treated in a more dehumanized manner. It can hurt the institution, which gets less than optimal performance from its employees and has to struggle with the disruptive problems of absenteeism and high turnover. It can hurt the caregiver's family, who experience more domestic strife and find an emotional gulf opening up between them. Indeed, the costs of burnout for all of society are clearly too high.

THE PERSONAL PRICE OF CARING

The emotional exhaustion of burnout may be accompanied by physical exhaustion as well. People report feeling tired and run-down, finding it hard to get up in the morning to face a new day. This tiredness comes from tension—the individual is wound up tight, unable to relax or sleep well at night. Insomnia may become a problem if continuous emotional tension prevents the person from unwinding enough to fall asleep or sleep deeply. Bad dreams and nightmares may begin to disturb his or her rest; sleepless nights of worry and of nagging, unnamed fears that "something" will go wrong occur more often.

Being chronically tired and tense can make you more susceptible to illness, and, indeed, people experiencing burnout mention the colds that linger too long and the headaches that do not go away. Decline in health can be exacerbated by poor eating habits—all too often, people under pressure may skip meals, eat on the run, or use the lunch hour to catch up on work. For some of them psychosomatic symptoms develop. Ulcers can occur, and neck and back problems are a frequent complaint.

> "On the way home from my first day on the job," said one prison guard, "I realized that my neck hurt. The muscles were tight, and that caused me to have a headache. Perspiration was heavier than normal. Later on, I noticed that my neck and shoulders would begin to get stiff and sore and painful just before I went to the prison—and it would last until I got home again." Some time afterward he reported, "My neck only hurts a little now, but the ringing in my ears has become more pronounced."

To cope with these physical problems, the burned-out provider may turn to tranquilizers, drugs, or alcohol. Having a drink before doing some stressful work, having a drink after the stressful encounter is over, having a drink to blot out the unpleasant memories and tensions of the day can become standard operating procedure for providers. In one school the morning announcements on payday would indicate where the faculty "rugby team" was having its match—in actuality, this was a code for where the drinking bout would be that evening to celebrate surviving another month. Similarly, tranquilizers are frequently used by providers who want to unwind and relax. They may also use some sort of stimulant or "upper" to get themselves going when they start their workday, and to keep themselves going they may rely on vast amounts of coffee. Aspirin is taken more often to fight off the pain of headaches, and the use of other medications to handle illnesses can also increase.

Each of these solutions for stress and illness has the potential for being abused. Drinking may shift from occasional to frequent, seriously impairing job performance. The cop having trouble with booze can pose a major hazard, as illustrated in the case of James. An alcoholic doctor or nurse clearly cannot provide good medical care.

> Helen, [a] recovered alcoholic nurse, now in her fourth year of sobriety, said she started to drink while working with a team of heavy drinkers in a cardiac operating room. "I fell right in with them," she said. "I loved to socialize with them after work. We had a ball." After several years of daily drinking accompanied by Valium pills, Helen said she began to have tremors at 5 P.M. every day. Her hands shook so badly, she said, that she was no longer able to scrub for operations or write reports about them, and instead had to work as a circulating nurse in the operating room.[2]

The touchy issue of alcoholism among professional helpers is only beginning to be recognized and acknowledged as a serious problem.

Like alcohol, tranquilizers and other drugs can be used excessively to the point of abuse. People who depend on pills to get going and to slow down can truly be considered drug addicts. Because of the body's adjusting tolerance for drugs, the person who uses sleeping pills for insomnia finds that over time ever-increasing amounts are needed to fall asleep. A drug problem can be even more serious if the provider has access to drugs in the course of his or her work.

> Herbert Freudenberger, who has written about his own and others' experiences with burnout in free clinics, makes this observation: "An irony that I have observed is that the burnt-out person who is working among drug addicts begins himself to become something of a con man as he 'requisitions' the pills from the institution's pharmacy and doctors."[3]

Physical health is not the only thing affected by burnout—*psychological* health is also involved. One phase of the burnout syndrome is a sense of reduced personal accomplishment and a loss of self-esteem. Providers begin to feel badly about themselves—about the kind of people they are and about the kind of job they have done or should have done. A visa officer says that she has become a "real bitch" as a result of her work and is saddened by this change in herself. A high school principal says he has used up all of his ideas and has become bitter. A mother says she feels guilty about spending less time with her children or yelling at them for no good reason. A former social worker says he began to despise himself for despising everyone else and that he finally quit his job and began seeing a psychiatrist because "I couldn't take myself anymore."

Feeling badly about oneself may lead to doing badly on the job—thus providing further evidence of one's lack of competence and self-worth. A tendency toward self-blame can lead people to tear themselves apart psychologically and can be a factor in further self-destructive behavior. In the end, providers who are down on themselves often pull away from other people, becoming isolates and nonparticipants. Then they are all alone in the trenches—an awfully frightening place to be.

A breakdown in self-esteem is a central characteristic of depression. This mood disorder is often a reaction to a sense of loss or a failure of some kind. In the case of burned-out helpers, the loss may be of original ideals or of "good people" to work with. Or the helpers may feel they have failed at their work or have failed to live up to their own standards. Depression may or may not interfere with the helper's work, depending on its degree of severity. However, the often-found relationship of depression to other problems, such as alcoholism, drug abuse, and suicide makes it a disorder deserving of serious attention and treatment.

> Available statistics show that the suicide rate is high for several people-work professions, including police, physicians, psychiatrists, and dentists. Although only a few cops actually "swallow their gun," their number may still be more than those cops who are killed in the line of duty. In 1976 about 480 New York police officers (2 percent of the force) were involved in gunplay. None of them was killed. However, five officers died by their own hand. They are the known "successful suicides" in one of the most stressful occupations.

Burnout can also affect psychological well-being in another way. The person who feels emotionally exhausted and has a growing dislike of people is too easily irritated. Even the most minor frustration can provoke an immediate response of anger. This anger not only increases negative feelings about others, but it feeds into an attitude of seething suspicion and mounting paranoia. The helper begins to believe that everybody is out to make trouble for him or her, deliberately making life difficult.

In addition, the provider may begin to feel omnipotent—that he or she knows everything and has seen it all before—"no one can run anything by *me.*" This may represent a last-ditch effort to stave off feelings of weakness, vulnerability, or failure. To convince themselves (and others) that they are strong and invulnerable, providers may take chances and expose themselves to risks, both on the job and off. Some risks may be lethal, others just the final failure experience before burnout is total. The problems associated with this sense of omnipotence and invulnerability are illustrated in the experience of staff members of alternative drug clinics.

> With these feelings of omnipotence, another real danger manifests itself—risk-taking. The burnt-out person will begin to take risks too readily. He begins, for example, to place himself in counseling situations that might be much too dangerous for one person to handle alone. He begins to think he can handle a speed freak, for example, all by himself in an apartment away from the clinic. Or, as happened in one instance, go out, late at night, to an abandoned parking lot to meet with an addict he hardly knew, who had called and dared him to come out and get him in for help. . . . I have noticed that the risk-taking behavior may even sometimes border on the lunatic. It has often appeared to me that the "crazy" behavior of the burnt-out person has something in it of a necessity. He seems to *need* to do something tht is out of his routine, even if what he does borders on the crazy—it is at least different.[4]

Psychological problems such as these should be treated through counseling or therapy of some kind. Unfortunately (and ironically) some professional helpers are among the people least likely to seek help for themselves. For example, doctors are notoriously reluctant to ask for aid, and the problems involved in obtaining treatment for the "impaired physician" are only now being recognized.[5] Mental health workers may avoid needed therapy because it would imply that they themselves are not mentally healthy–and *they*, after all, are the ones who should be. People who are supposed to have all the answers and be able to help everyone else may view their own difficulties as a sign of incompetence or failure. Thus, ministers may be loath to admit they need help because they fear the loss of trust and respect among their parishioners and because they may not know where to turn. Police are often unwilling to avail themselves of counseling or psychiatric services because to do so would be a sign of weakness and unreliability and an admission that they are really crazy–"psycho cops." The prevailing view among many police officers is that "if you need to see a shrink, you shouldn't be a cop in the first place."

THE PRICE OTHER PEOPLE PAY

The person who burns out is not the only one to suffer ill effects; many others are also singed by burnout. Recipients of the individual's care or services, co-workers, family, and friends–all these people can testify to the costs that the person's burnout has had for *them* as well.

Burnout and the Job

Perhaps the most visible impact of burnout is the change in people's work performance. Basically, they do a less good job. Motivation is down, frustration is up, and an unsympathetic, "don't-give-a-damn" attitude predominates. They don't take care in making their judgments, and they don't care as much about the outcome. They "go by the book" and are stale rather than innovative and fresh. They give the bare minimum rather than giving their all, and sometimes they give nothing at all. As one longtime schoolteacher said, "My motto is, 'The more they ask, the less I do.' "

With increased burnout, there is an increase in "processing the work load," in treating people as objects and not as fellow human beings. To some extent, this asocial view is promoted by the professional tendency to treat "problems" rather than people. Hospital staff will refer to "the coronary" who was just admitted; legal service attorneys identify their clients as "my SSI disability," "my truth-in-lending," and so forth. Labeling people by their problem is done for two reasons. First of all, the problem *is* the basis for the helping relationship. Second, labeling protects the confidentiality of the helper-recipient relationship by not revealing the recipient's personal identity. However, such labeling becomes part of the caregiver's mental structure, out of which emerges a dehumanized view of the recipients. In a letter to the editor of the *Journal of the American Medical Association,* Dr. John W. Goppelt points out the detrimental consequences of identifying patients by their illness:

> Some psychiatrists have objected to the practice of referring to persons by their diseases or their diseased parts. Internists and surgeons have been advised not to speak of the gallbladder in bed 3, the appendix in bed 1, or the pulmonary embolism in bed 2. Physicians have been urged, correctly as I believe, to attend to the whole person, but we psychiatrists are in the habit of speaking of this schizophrenic or that manic-depressive or that obsessive-compulsive. It might be well if we were to remind ourselves that mental illness is not the whole person but only a part of that person, and that if we persist in equating a person's mental illness with him, we run the risk of unwittingly assuming a condescending attitude toward him and the further risk of influencing other persons to assume the same attitude toward him.[6]

When caregivers view recipients more as "things" than as people, there are changes in the way they take care of them. Not only is the treatment of service more routinized, but the provider pays less attention to the recipient's human needs. Consequently, the provider may say or do things that are thoughtless, discourteous, or rude, and may display an insensitivity to the recipient's feelings. For example, after the death of their young son, the grieving parents met with a hospital staff person who smiled and said cheerily, "And where shall we send the little fella?" Clearly, the remark was highly inappropriate. Does it matter to the parents if it was not intentionally so?

> In another instance, a young woman was hospitalized following a stroke that had left her legs paralyzed. When her husband came to visit, he found that she was routinely being spoon-fed her meals by the nurses—even though nothing was wrong with her hands or arms. Although the nurses probably meant well, they were actually making the patient feel helpless, passive, infantile, and even less in control of her life. Unfortunately, when her husband objected and asked that she be allowed to feed herself, one of the nurses was angered by the criticism and retaliated with the threat of abandoning the patient: "Well, if you insist on making such a big issue over nothing, I'll see to it that she gets left alone altogether."

As burned-out helpers come to dislike the people they serve, callous and cruel remarks may be made deliberately. One New York social worker taunted a client who was trying to get child support payments by saying, "You need money, Mrs. W? Why don't you walk the streets?" A West Coast surgeon became enraged by the questions posed by a patient's sister and yelled at her, "If it weren't against the law, my fist would be in your mouth, and that would be one good way of closing it and shutting you up!" Teachers may begin to regard some of their students as "animals" or other lower forms of life.

Callous and dehumanized attitudes are often translated into callous and dehumanized behavior. Mental hospital staff may overuse drugs to calm patients and make them easier to manage. Physical force may be overused to control potentially violent patients, as illustrated by the recent case of an employee at California's Camarillo State Hospital, who choked a patient to death. Police may use excessive force when making an arrest. Guards in prisons and county jails may become so emotionally hardened and inured to the conditions that they will stand idly by as prisoners are subjected to beatings and sexual assaults. Medical staff may provide inhumane treatment not only to the patient but extend the discourtesy to the patient's family as well.

Instead of doing their work badly, many burned-out helpers do less of it. They avoid certain tasks ("I'm not the one who does that"). Or they simply spend less time with their patient or client by deliberately cutting down the length of the interview, instruction, or therapy session. As one psychiatric nurse put it, "Some patients are so frustrating to work with—I won't spend more than thirty minutes with any of them." In some instances the reduction in client contact is achieved more indirectly.

> The ready smile and the too quickly given statement, "I'm sure everything will be just fine," frequently amount only to an unrecognized but socially acceptable means of telling the patient that one is really not concerned with him as a human being in pain and difficulty. The "friendly and reassuring" pat on the back may also be employed as a polite means of pushing the patient out of the office.[7]

Professional caregivers may also avoid contact with recipients by spending more of their time talking and socializing with other staff members. In some mental hospitals at any given time the staff are more likely to be found inside their glass "cages" than circulating among the patients on the ward.

The emotional strain of working with many people can lead helpers to withdraw psychologically and have minimal contact with them. The helper is physically present but acts as if the other person were not. There is little eye contact, questions are answered with a mumble or grunt (if at all), and there is an avoidance of any body contact, such as handshakes or hugs. In some cases providers busy themselves with tasks that exclude the recipients from direct participation (as when a counselor stretches out the time it takes to complete necessary forms, forcing the client to sit and wait). Burned-out providers not only minimize their relationships with recipients, they may fantasize about "ideal" jobs in which few, if any, people exist. For instance, when I asked Bert G., a social worker, what job he would like to have most of all, he replied, "Well, I love art. And what I would love to do is work in a museum—all by myself, with no one around to bother me—cataloging paintings in the storage rooms. Just the paintings and me—that's all."

Over time, the burned-out provider will withdraw physically from the job. Coffee breaks become longer, lunch "hours" are more than sixty minutes, and the time to go home comes earlier in the working day. At one social welfare agency we learned never to schedule interviews for Friday afternoons because no

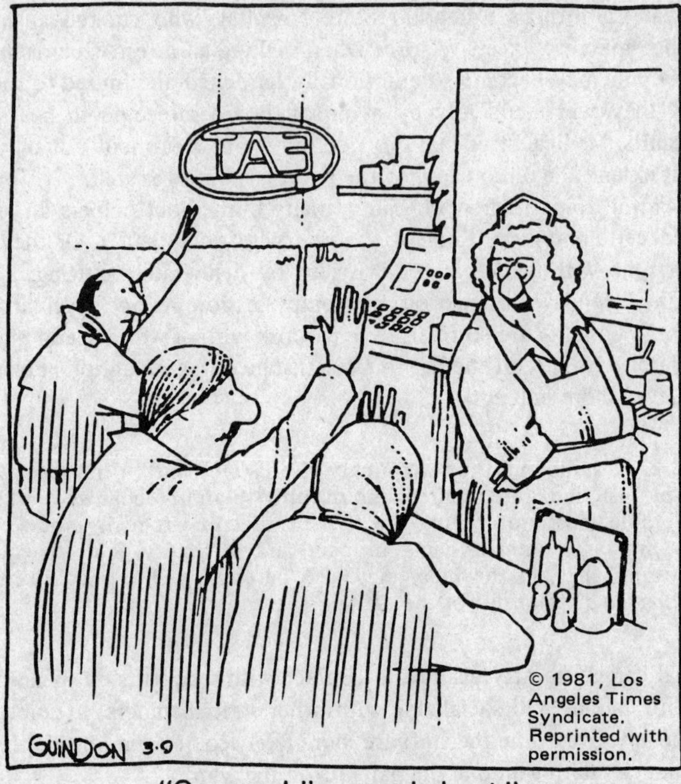

"Go away! I'm peopled out."

staff people would be there—not because they were making home visits with their clients but because they had simply gone to their own homes. Absenteeism is more prevalent with burnout, and some staff people routinely take their maximum sick leave.

At some point the helping work may become too much and the provider quits. "I have friends who had such overwhelming demands on their time and on their emotions that they just stopped and refused to do any more work," said one psychiatric social worker. A welfare administrator in the Southwest told about his burnout after several years of directing War on Poverty programs: "I found myself less able to handle my emotions, but rather than cutting myself off from my emotions, I quit." Service and claims representatives in Social Security offices who were suffering from burnout were most likely to say that they planned to leave their job within a year.[8]

The link between burnout and turnover often appears early. Two years (give or take a year) is most frequently cited as the first critical point at which burnout will lead people to quit and get out. In some cases, the person leaves the field entirely, taking a new job in a totally different line of work. A psychiatric nurse becomes a carpenter, or a counselor turns to farming. They swear they will never return to their original occupation with its crush of people and emotional demands.

More often, providers who quit move to a different job within their field, typically one in administration. Not only do administrators have more prestige, power, and pay, they have less direct contact with clients. Many social workers who return to school for an advanced degree are quite frank about their need to reduce their involvement with people. Said one, "We're going back to school to become administrators or teachers or whatever—so that our client contact will be limited, and we won't be forced to become callous in order to stay sane." Susan T., the poverty lawyer described in Chapter 2, left legal services to become director of admissions at a law school. "I have a lovely office," she said, "where it's quiet, and I can close the door anytime I want to. Most of the people I deal with are in the form of application folders—pieces of paper, rather than flesh-and-blood human beings. And I like it that way." Thus, the move into administration is often an attempt to escape from the emotional strain of people work.

> It is our impression that many psychiatrists and clinical psychologists escape from the front-line trenches of clinical practice into the relative security of administration, teaching and research. Most active case work appears to be done by the very young who are still idealistic, hopeful and enthusiastic. The burden of endless case handling of hard-core patients exerts its toll in feelings of ineffectuality, impotence and frustration. Some clinicians choose suicide or to leave the field. An honorable escape lies in promotion to nonclinical duties where one can rest on his laurels, and gain greater prestige and influence.[9]

Burnout and the Family

The detrimental effects of burnout do not stop when the professional helper calls it a day and heads for home. Burnout can damage his or her personal life as well. The cynical dislike of people and the emotional exhaustion may arise from the job, but their impact may be strongly felt by the helper's family and friends.

The provider who is emotionally exhausted will come home feeling tense, upset, and physically tired. A lot of time will be spent bitching and complaining about the job. Lacking the emotional energy to handle everyday hassles calmly, the helper at home is irritable and impatient, a *problem* that the family has to learn how to deal with. Said the husband of one social worker,

> When she comes home, she's just steaming. She rants and raves about everything, and I try to be supportive and help her unwind, but finally I don't want to hear it anymore and I tell her to quit bugging me. So she accuses me of not being sympathetic, and I say why can't she just relax and forget about the job, and she says she *can't* forget about it because she's dealing with people's lives, and so on and so forth. So now we're both pretty tense and picking at each other and certainly not in the mood to make love or have a good time together.

The increased fighting and bickering can lead to family squabbles and serious marital conflict. This domestic discord is often not recognized as stemming from the stress of the job—instead, it is attributed to something that has gone wrong in the marital relationship ("I guess we don't love each other anymore"). Separation or divorce are then possible outcomes. As one correctional officer put it when we were talking about the pressures of working in prison, "None of my three wives understood."

When the work drains all your emotional energy, you are less able and willing to give to others outside of the work—even if those "others" are presumably the most significant and cherished people in your life. "I don't want to hear another problem or another human voice—I just want some peace and quiet," is a common refrain. Unfortunately, this desire for solitude often comes at the expense of family and friends. *They* are the ones who are shut out while you recoup your emotional strength. Said one teacher, "My energies were flowing too heavily in one direction (the job) for me to be able to give much time and effort to our marriage. It had never been a perfect relationship, but it might have worked—if I had been able to bring more to it. At the beginning of the sixth school year, my husband and I separated."

Unable to get involved with his or her family, the burned-out provider will see them first get angry and make greater demands for attention. Family members may be jealous of the care and attention that the provider gives to recipients, and not to them. They will then begin to withdraw, feeling hurt and neglected. According to the son of one minister, "My father spends a lot of time working with people who are needy or troubled, but when he comes home he just disappears into the den. He's always there when other people want him, but he's not there for me. I know he's considered a great man, but he's not a great father."

Compounding the problems of emotional withdrawal is the tendency for some providers to refuse to discuss their job with their family.

> "I never tell my wife what I'm doing—never," one police officer said. "And we're always having conflicts about this. She comes home from work, and all she does all night long is tell me about the kids she teaches and what went on in school. And she says, 'You never tell me about what you do, you never talk to me about it.' Because I don't *want* to talk to her

about it. I don't want her to know what I do here—it would just make it worse."

This refusal to "talk shop" is usually justified in terms of protecting one's family from the grim realities of the job. "It would upset them to hear about the patients' psychotic episodes or suicide attempts," said one psychiatric technician, "so I don't bother to tell them." However, the providers may really be trying to protect *themselves* from the stress of their work. They don't want to relive the day's events and reexperience the feelings they had. Ralph V., a prison psychologist, described it this way:

> I've told my wife *never* to ask me about what goes on in the prison. I say, "If I ever think there's something you should know about the prison, then I'll tell you—but don't ever ask me. I've already gone through the day once, and I don't want to go through it again." Sometimes I'll see a new guard coming to work tired and troubled, and I'll say to him, "I bet you've been going home every night and telling your wife about everything you do here," and he'll say, "Yeah, you're right—how did you know?" And I'll say, "Here's a piece of good advice—don't tell her about it anymore. Ever. That's the only way you'll survive with this job."

Ralph believes in the personal advantages of not sharing the job with one's spouse. But it also poses serious disadvantages for the marital relationship because it creates barriers to an open, trusting, sharing partnership.

Although the helper may not actively talk about the job at home, it can still have an insidious and powerful impact on family life. Family members may be under constant scrutiny and pressured to be perfect, with no problems of their own. "After all, the child of a (minister, policeman, judge) shouldn't be getting into trouble." Contact with family members is reduced and family activities are disrupted whenever the provider works overtime or has unusual working hours, as with night shifts in a hospital or weekend police patrols. Similarly, the person who brings home work from the office or who spends off hours in professional activities (such as breakfast conferences or evening staff meetings) is making major cuts in his or her personal home life. In some cases, there is virtually no personal life at all, since the job begins to occupy all one's waking hours. Recall the case of William Van Buskirk, the high school principal described in Chapter 3, who worked seven days and five nights a week at his job, and whose marriage eventually broke up.

The provider's personal life is also disrupted when he or she is "on call." Not knowing when (or if) an emergency will arise, but having to be ready to respond to it, the provider cannot fully relax and unwind after a hard day's work. Even one's sleep may be interrupted (as in the incident with Robert T., the social worker described at the beginning of this chapter). Leisure activities are limited or even curtailed. Some providers are "on call" only for certain periods, such as weekends or two nights during the week. Others are "on call" all the time, twenty-four hours a day—parents being a prime example. Providers in private practice may also be subject to continuous demands.

> For many psychiatrists, a drawback of going into private practice is that the job intrudes too much in personal life. As one psychiatrist, Veronica C., put it, "Every time I hear the telephone ring at night, I think, 'Oh God—I hope it's not a patient.' At times it seems as if I can't even get away from my patients' problems for some peace and quiet for myself. When I worked at the hospital, there wasn't the same problem because when I went home for the day, another shift came on—and so I could relax in the evenings because I knew that if any of the patients needed help, there was someone else there to provide it."

Some providers may put themselves "on call" voluntarily at first, by making their telephone number available to their clients or students or whoever—"If you have a problem, feel free to call me anytime." However, as the calls become too frequent, especially at odd hours (some people *do* call at "anytime"), the provider may become hostile toward recipients and will soon drop the open-telephone policy altogether.

A more subtle, but no less serious, way in which the professional helper's job interferes with private life is when he or she cannot shake the professional role. The caregiver acts toward family and friends as if they were clients or patients. For instance, therapists may begin to "treat" their personal acquaintances, often without recognizing that they are doing so. Helpers who are always "on call" find it especially hard to shed their professional demeanor. As an example, a cop is always expected to be a cop, even when off duty.

> To survive on the job, a policeman develops a tough skin. This emotional cool, suspiciousness, and sense of caution cannot be taken off and put away as easily as his uniform. They become second nature to him, an integral part of relating to *all* people, including his family. Unwittingly, he becomes more tough and aggressive when dealing with his wife and kids, questions them more often, appears to mistrust them, is more rigid in deciding what's "wrong" or "right," and is less emotionally involved with his family. The wife of a California police officer summed it up this way: "I can't understand how seemingly normal husbands turn into such 'machos.' Arguments end in 'Because I said so.' Our children feel as though they really can't discuss problems with their father because he relates in terms of the law and logic, and not the emotions involved. Sometimes I feel that if I don't do what he wants, I'll be arrested."[10]

The negative, cynical feelings about people that develop with burnout are not limited to those individuals one encounters on the job. They become more pervasive and are the basis of a more permanently soured view of humanity. "It's a feeling of total disgust with people," said one social worker. "Let's face it, everyone is as rotten as the next person–myself included." Police who constantly see people at their worst and have to deal with the aftermath of such terrible events as rape, murder, and assault find it easy to begin believing that everyone is basically evil. Sadly, this grim attitude about fellow human beings becomes internalized and relatively resistant to change. The experience of Marjorie W., the Social Security service representative we met in Chapter 3, illustrates this point. She was eventually able to obtain a noninterviewing position and is now under less emotional strain. Her husband reports that she is not as grouchy or nervous as she used to be and that she does not snap at people so much. "But," he said thoughtfully, "she's still very cynical about people, very untrusting–that hasn't changed at all, and it's been several years now." Here, perhaps, is the most devastating legacy of burnout–a permanent hardening of the human heart.

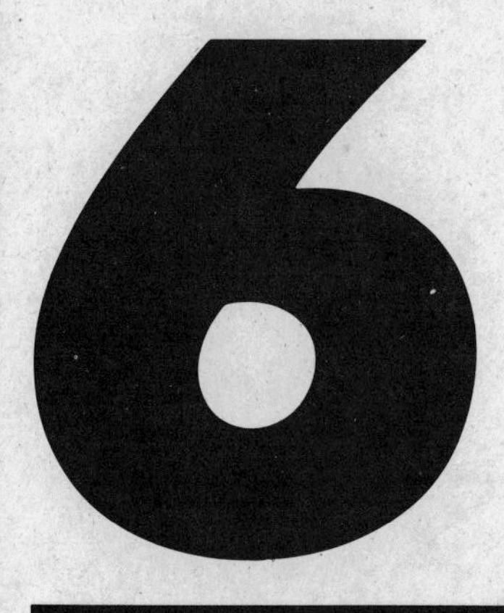

HOW TO HANDLE BURNOUT: DOING IT ON YOUR OWN

Sometimes I just feel like giving up. When that happens, I'll tell a patient, "You know, I'm really frustrated right now. I feel like I'm not getting anywhere, so why don't we wait until later to talk." Then I try to get out of the problem for awhile. I'll talk to somebody else, or I'll sit in the office and do a lot of paperwork. Or I'll try to get assigned to medications for the day. Some days I'm with the patients the whole time; other days, I schedule less contact with them. I don't come back on days off—I really try to get away. It's important to be aware of when things are getting out of hand and I'm getting emotionally wiped out. Then I talk with some other people about what's happening to me, and I just lay low for a few days.

Jennifer B., psychiatric nurse

After school, I work as a gymnastics coach. This gives me contact with students that is different from teaching, so it helps me see them in a different light and can offset some of the daily frustrations. Plus it gives me a chance to exercise, work off tension, and keep in good physical condition. During the summer I get as far away from teaching as possible. I look forward to that summer job: lifeguard, house painter, salesman, or whatever. Sometimes, that job becomes a year-round vocation. Moonlighting is often a financial necessity because teachers' salaries are pretty inadequate. But, more important, it is an emotional survival technique."

Roger E., teacher

The costs of burnout can be high. Both the provider and the recipient of care are affected negatively by it, as are other people in their lives and the helping institutions that help less well. Sadly, some of these costs represent coping techniques gone awry. The helper has tried to reduce the stress of burnout, perhaps by taking alcohol or drugs, or by getting away from people, but these actions have had as many, or more, detrimental consequences as beneficial ones.

Fortunately, there are more constructive approaches to coping with burnout. Each of them, in its own way, tackles one or more of the three major aspects of the burnout syndrome: (a) it may reduce the emotional strains of people work; (b) it may offset the negative, depersonalized views of people; and (c) it may boost the individual's sense of personal accomplishment and self-esteem. Each approach requires patience and practice to be used successfully. There are no quick and easy solutions to the problem of burnout. Each of them has to be adapted to the specific job and home situation of the individual provider. For example, the person in private practice will utilize a social technique differently than someone working as part of a team. Finally, not all coping techniques are for all people—what works best for one person may be less successful for someone else. Some activities may not be feasible in a particular job setting, and some may be rejected as a matter of personal choice. What is important is that all of these approaches can help in the battle against burnout, so let's consider seriously the potential merits of each of them. You can then decide which ones are best for you in your work context.

Coping can occur at several different levels—individual, social, and institutional. At the individual level are actions that you can take on your own. Social coping techniques are those that require the joint efforts of several people, such as your co-workers. Coping techniques at the institutional level refer to policies and administrative actions that can help the staff deal with emotional stress. In this chapter I will cover only individual strategies. I will discuss a range of social and institutional approaches in the next chapter.

INDIVIDUAL COPING

What can one person do about burnout? A lot, as it turns out. Some of these coping techniques involve your style of work, while others focus on your general life-style.

Working Smarter instead of Working Harder

When people are overwhelmed by the job they are doing, a common response is to work even harder in an attempt to catch up and get back in control of things. They do the same things they have been doing all along, only they do more of them. For providers, that means seeing more people with problems, spending more time with them, doing more paperwork, and so on. However, working harder often contributes to the stress of burnout, rather than relieving it. Seeing more people increases the possibility of emotional exhaustion, and spending more time on their problems heightens the development of a cynical dislike of human beings. And to the extent that it is difficult or even impossible *ever* to catch up with the work, a sense of frustration and personal failure are likely to occur.

Working harder, then, is not the best solution for coping with burnout—but working smarter is. By "working smarter" I mean making changes in the way you handle your job so that you are less stressed and more efficient. If we use the analogy of driving a car, when going up a steep hill it is better to shift down to a lower gear than just to give it more gas at high gear. There are many possible ways of shifting gears in your work, rather than always being in automatic drive.

SETTING REALISTIC GOALS Professional helpers are often striving for noble ideals—fighting injustice, making the world a better place to live in, bringing health and happiness to all, and so forth. While there is much to praise in such ideals, they also have drawbacks. Ideals are highly abstract and refer to vague and general goals that are virtually impossible to achieve within one's lifetime. These characteristics of noble ideals can pose problems for a provider when ideals are all he or she has to guide the direction of work, because then, no matter how hard the person works, each day is doomed to be a failure. Either the person cannot tell whether or not any progress has been made toward that abstract ideal ("Is my client *really* better off, happier, more well-adjusted?") or the ideal is never reached ("No matter what I do, there is still poverty, injustice, sickness").

This is not to knock the impossible dream. But impossible dreams are only good motivators if the pathway toward them is marked by specific signposts. A person needs to know if progress *has* been made, if something *has* been accomplished, if steps *have* been taken that will make the dream a reality someday. If the ideal is not to be a source of frustration and failure, it must be accompanied by concrete subgoals that are clearly possible to achieve. These realistic goals are often not provided for the caregiver—rather, the person must discover how to make them explicit in the process of defining them.

In practical terms, this means that you have to work out a list of specific accomplishments that you can shoot for on a given day, a given month—even for the year. For example, "By the end of the week, I'll try to complete the file on Mrs. X, visit the Y family, see five new clients"; or "I'll spend an hour with this patient and get her to clarify what she expects from her visits with her family," and so forth. The key word here is *specific*—the possible accomplishments have to be well defined in concrete terms. If they refer to specific behaviors, rather than general abstractions, then they are clearly "do-able." Compare "talking to Mr. A about taking a new medication, suggesting to Mr. A that he enroll in a weight-reduction program, setting up a return appointment for Mr. A" with "helping Mr. A with his heart problem." With the specific goals, the health practitioner will have accomplished something by the end of the day or week and will be more likely to see some progress in the care provided. The abstract goal, however, is less likely to be accomplished soon—and, in fact, may never be realized completely (suppose Mr. A continues to have heart problems or fails to follow prescribed treatment). Note that the specific goals represent steps toward the more abstract ideal. By focusing on those steps, you can measure progress and feel a sense of accomplishment. If, however, you focus only on the end point, the result is more likely to be frustration, failure, and a feeling of "why can't I ever get anything done?"

Not only should these goals be specific, they should be *realistic* as well. By realistic, I mean that there must be a reasonable chance that you will actually be able to accomplish the goal. If the goal is virtually impossible to achieve, then you are doomed to failure. Setting realistic goals involves a recognition of your limitations as well as of your abilities.

> As an example, psychotherapists working with young cancer patients must realize that they cannot prevent some of them from dying, but that they can improve their lives in specifiable ways. "From time to time I must remind myself that if I am successful my patients will be more comfortable, less anxious, and communicate more effectively with the people close to them. I have no influence over their malignancy and no responsibility for its outcome."[1]

DOING THE SAME THING DIFFERENTLY When a helper feels helpless—trapped, in a rut, powerless—burnout is more likely to set in. Helplessness can produce frustration and anger, and these twin demons, in turn, can leave the helper emotionally exhausted and hostile. Handling burnout at this level means conquering the sense of helplessness. By choosing to do things in different ways and varying your work routine, you can get out of that rut and feel more in control of your job. Not only can some major tasks be done differently, such as adopting a new mode of therapy for a client, but ordinary, everyday tasks can also be handled in new ways—even such mundane things as answering the telephone, greeting patients, or starting a class. Consider the new response of a substitute teacher to the old problem of getting a class going:

> It is a given, of course, that at the sight of a "sub," students develop full bladders, empty tablets and blunt pencils. They simply can't start class

> unless they can go to the bathroom, borrow paper and sharpen their pencils. . . . If you tell a kid he or she can't sharpen a pencil, it's a cinch that pencil will wind up playing taps on your eardrums. I took a cue from Neil Diamond, who lets his fans blast away at will with their flash-cubes during one, and only one, song of his concerts. I devoted the first two minutes of a fifth grade class to nothing but pencil-sharpening. Furious scrambling. Grinding. Cranking. But in the end it saved time and my sanity.[2]

To be effective in doing things differently, you first have to figure out which aspects of the job can be changed or varied and which cannot. There are bound to be some things that are fixed and not subject to change, such as certain institutional rules, for example. It is best to avoid putting your energy into changing these things until you have proven to yourself that you have learned how to modify less formidable aspects of your job. Instead, focus on what *can* be modified, varied, shifted around, or handled at your own discretion. For example, you might be able to reshuffle your contact hours with clients—by doing all your counseling in the morning, breaking it up into several sessions interspersed with paperwork, or scheduling your most difficult clients just before your lunch break. Or you might find ways to share your most distressing work with others, or to do it less often by cutting down the less essential parts of it. Or you might try to explain things to recipients in a new way—using different examples, having groups of recipients meet together instead of singly, and so forth.

The benefit of doing things differently is sometimes purely psychological. The helper has a greater sense of autonomy and personal freedom, even while handling the same old problems. To illustrate, a nurse may give the same medical care to patients as she would have anyway, but she may feel more in control of her work by having *chosen* which patients to see first or which patients to spend a little extra time with in pleasant conversation. The person who *chooses* is the actor and director in the drama of life, instead of part of the passive audience who merely react to someone else's plot and stage directions.

In other instances, doing things differently may go beyond changing one's self-concept. It may, in fact, alleviate a source of stress. The accepted, standard way of handling a task may be ineffective or the inadvertent cause of additional emotional strain, and thus a change may actually improve the situation as well as provide an opportunity for personal control.

> Donald K. was a social worker whose clients were mostly elderly people. Many of them were severely depressed by their life situation, and the standard procedure was to give them a referral to a medical doctor for counseling. However, such referrals were not always easily made, and so Donald decided to bend the rule a bit and referred some of his clients to a psychologist instead. He then discovered that he was getting fewer complaints from those clients on return visits and fewer hassles from the doctors. Apparently, the doctors had viewed Donald's clients as "crocks" who were wasting the doctors' time and medical skills because they were

not physically ill. The type of counseling provided by the psychologist was more in line with the clients' needs, and so Donald's unofficial change in institutional policy actually solved an unrecognized problem.

BREAKING AWAY The stress of people work can be reduced by arranging intermittent breaks or rest periods. Such breaks serve as emotional breathers, allowing you to relax, "take five," and get a little psychological distance from a particular problem. Rude or angry remarks made in the heat of frustration are less likely to occur if you have had a chance to cool off emotionally.

One type of break is a short pause that is built in to your contact with people. Although brief, this is a "pause that refreshes" because you have enough time to slow down, regain calm, stop a situation that is getting out of hand, and start all over again. Sometimes the pause is explicitly stated as such. For example, one therapist reported that if the therapy hour was not going well, he would say to the client, "Wait a minute—let me think about what you've just said." Then he *would* take a minute or two to sit silently, eyes closed or covered by his hand, while he tried to relax and figure out what to say to get the discussion back on the track. In other instances, the pause occurs in the guise of some aspect of the work routine. A college counselor who says, "Just a moment—I'll have to get your file from the next room" may be using that short trek to collect her thoughts and count to ten before returning to handle the complaint of the irate student. Short pauses can also be inserted between contact with different recipients. Cutting a thirty-minute interview to twenty-five does not change its content very much, but it may give you a chance to close the door and relax briefly before seeing the next person.

Official breaks from work, such as coffee breaks and the lunch hour, are standard procedure in most organizations. These can be ideal opportunities for emotional recharging, but unfortunately they are sometimes misused in ways that aggravate burnout. Most commonly, people continue to work during their breaks, catching up on paperwork, making telephone calls, or doing some other chores. To go back to our automobile analogy, although these people are keeping their foot on the accelerator only lightly, they should be putting it on the brake. Whatever gains come from working around the clock are usually outweighed by the loss of energy and patience and by the increase in errors or poor judgments toward the end of the workday. It is far better to take advantage of these breaks and really get away from the pressures and demands of the helping role. When the lunch hour comes, leave the office and go for a walk, read a book, get together with friends, play cards, jog, listen to music, plan a sumptuous dinner, visit a local art gallery—indulge yourself. Harriet C., who worked twelve years as a college registrar and counselor, put it this way:

> I think coffee breaks and lunch period *away from the clients* are absolutely essential. I learned by experience that I came back to my desk

> rested and better able to "cope" because I had had that time away from the students, time behind a closed door, time to read the newspaper or just get away from the college for an hour. You need to feel you can escape at regular times and that there is at least one place where you can let down and be yourself, as a person, rather than the counselor or registrar or whatever.

In line with the recommendation to use your breaks wisely is the caution not to overdo overtime. Providers are often pressured to put in extra time—to schedule appointments before or after regular hours, to attend meetings during lunch, to stay late or return in the evening to "catch up" on work, and so forth. In many cases, there is no compensation for such overtime, either in extra pay or time off. Consequently, providers are more likely to be emotionally exhausted and to feel hostility and resentment toward their recipients and co-workers.

When things get particularly difficult or frustrating, it is important to be able to withdraw completely from the situation. One possibility is not to work for awhile—to cancel appointments, take a day of sick leave, stretch out the lunch hour. However, such reactive "escapes" have the disadvantage of suddenly reducing service or care, since no one else may be able to take over your responsibilities easily. Furthermore, you are likely to feel guilty about the recipients who are not receiving attention, thereby adding to, rather than ameliorating, your burden of emotional exhaustion.

A more positive form of withdrawal is a work change, or "downshift."[3] Downshifts are not breaks from work in the sense of rest periods or time away from the job. Rather, they are opportunities for the helper to do some other, less emotionally stressful work while someone else takes over the responsibilities for recipients.

> For example, in one psychiatric ward that I studied, the nurses knew that if they were having a rough day, they could arrange to do something else besides work directly with patients. "There are times on the ward when I know that I'm not as capable of giving that much of myself," said one of them, "so I'll sit in the office and do a lot of paperwork. The way our schedule, is, it gives you the opportunity to do that. You can withdraw and choose to attend meetings for a while. Or you can ask to get assigned to medications, so that you spend the entire day in the medicine room. Then, the only time you see patients is when you're calling on them for medicines." In this system, when one nurse took a downshift, the other nurses would cover for her and continue to provide adequate patient care.

TAKING THINGS LESS PERSONALLY The emotional exhaustion of burnout escalates when you get overly involved with people—taking on their problems as your own, reacting to negative comments as if they were personal insults, and so on. When things begin to get this intense, you should try to stand back and look at the situation in more abstract and intellectual terms. By "objectifying" the situation, you are less likely to get emotionally entangled in it. For example, as we saw in Chapter 2, a psychiatric technician faced with an abusive mental patient will try to understand first if the anger is part of the patient's disorder rather than a personal attack on himself. The same sort of process happens with parents as their child passes through different developmental stages. Rather than interpreting the child's temper tantrum or fear of strangers as a sign that "I'm not a good parent" or "My child doesn't really love me," the parent will react by saying, "It's just a phase she (or he) is going through."

Emotional overinvolvement can also be reduced if you do not "take home" people's problems. By leaving your work *at* work and not reliving it again at home, the emotional stress is confined to a smaller part of your life.

> Eric C., a social worker in child welfare, stated that if he did not leave his work at the office, he could hardly stand to face his own children. Likewise, when he was at work he could not think of his family because he would then overidentify and overemphathize with his clients and treat their misfortunes as his own—an emotional experience that he could not handle repeatedly.

Several therapists reported a shift in their orientation toward clients' struggles from "their pain is my pain" to "their pain is their pain." Although they still cared about their clients' progress and helped in whatever way they could, they realized that they did not need to experience the clients' feelings to be effective therapists.

Caring for Oneself, as well as for Others

Helping and caring for other people is highly demanding work. Meeting these demands without falling victim to burnout can best be done by people who are strong, both in body and spirit, and who make sure they stay that way. You must be in good shape yourself truly to give unto others; thus, taking care of Number One is an essential prerequisite for taking care of Numbers Two, Three, Four, and so on. Techniques that promote physical and psychological well-being can do much to offset the negative costs of burnout.

ACCENTUATING THE POSITIVE Helping relationships have a negative bias. All too often problems take precedence to the point where people focus only on what is wrong and forget about what is right. An effective way to counter this negative bias is to emphasize actively what is good or pleasant or satisfying about your contact with others. Taking the good along with the bad makes the bad less total and overwhelming. Frustrations and failures can be put into perspective when balanced by satisfactions and successes.

Accentuating the positive can take many forms. At one level, it means paying more attention to your accomplishments—the minor ones as well as the major ones. Having an interesting conversation, sharing a joke, helping someone with directions, and so forth, are positive achievements that should not be ignored or underestimated. When the day is done, you ought to take time to count up all the things that went well and to bask in the glow of that knowledge—rather than simply to agonize over the things that fell short.

In line with this approach is the reevaluation of your work to find positive aspects about it that may have been previously unrecognized.

> Burton K., a marriage and family counselor, reports that he now views therapy as replenishment. "I feel I get replenished in therapy because I also get from my clients—genuine emotions, which I now see as an act of caring, trust, giving, even when they give me anger or their sadness. That human sharing replenishes me. I don't feel used if people cry or hold me or are angry with me, even though I may be used."

This strategy of looking for the good in one's work is related to the "half-full versus half-empty" personal style that I discussed in Chapter 4. The "half-full" style is a deliberate attempt to accentuate the positive—even in situations where you might think there is precious little to be enthusiastic about.

> Dr. Robert Veninga of the University of Minnesota illustrates how we might make the most of even a very routine job. He cites the bus driver whose route is a three-block link between University Hospitals and a parking lot. "I observed what he's doing. Rather than just moving the bus from point to point he's obviously made a commitment to helping people, either by waiting for them or directing them to where they want to go. Somebody can say driving a bus is not fulfilling, but if you talked to this guy he'd probably tell you he meets all kinds of interesting people every day and feels he is helping some of them."[4]

Two things are noteworthy about this bus driver. First, his focus is on the pleasant and rewarding aspects of his work as opposed to the unpleasant and tedious ones. Second, he actively elicits positive reactions from his passengers by talking about interesting topics and doing nice things for them. He does not simply wait for good things to happen—he *makes* them happen as well. The deliberate inclusion of some positive moments in your contact with people can offset the negative biases and experiences that arise from dealing with people's problems. The jokes, compliments, and "small talk" that make up these positive moments are often irrelevant to the problem itself, but they can make management of the problem a less debilitating process.

> Connie S., a physical therapist, says that she often converses with patients during the therapy sessions. "We talk about their family, or their hobbies, or the latest football scores, or a new movie, or the weather, or whatever. Because I see patients many times, rather than just once or twice, I have many conversations with them—so we really get acquainted and develop good feelings for each other. When you learn to know patients as indi-

vidual people, it is very difficult to think of them as amputees, strokes, and hip fractures."

The earlier advice to do things differently applies here as well. Restructuring a situation is another way of transforming it into a more positive experience.

For Margo N., a teacher in a preschool, lunch was always spent in the company of twenty rambunctious five-year-olds. How could this noontime meal become less a dreaded event and more of a delight? Suppose there were music, candlelight, quiet conversation, an attentive maître d'–that might be nice. So Margo took steps to change Classroom D into Café Dee during the lunch hour. One child is in charge of putting records on the phonograph, another puts flowers on the table, and Margo lights the candles. The maitre d' of the day announces the rules (civilities to be observed) and is responsible for reminding disruptive diners of that agreed upon code of conduct. One child serves the soup, and everyone waits for another one to say, "*Bon appétit*, now you may eat"–the ritual signal to begin the meal. Lunchtime in Café Dee has now become a very pleasant occasion–both for the teacher and the students.

Making good things happen also means making good feedback happen. Praise and thanks are not always forthcoming, even when your work has been good enough to deserve it. Appreciation is often absent because the work is taken for granted–it may not have occurred to the client or patient that some kind words would be welcome. In other cases, recipients may not give feedback because it is especially difficult for them to do so (and not because they are unappreciative). They may be very shy or fearful of authority, or they may have language problems of some kind. Therefore, you may have to be active in seeking out positive feedback, rather than passively awaiting (praying for) its possible arrival. In other words, ask for it! "If this helps you (solves the problem, makes you feel better), I would appreciate it if you would tell me"; "Let me know if this works out"; "I can do a better job for you if I know what you *like* about my work (as well as what you dislike)"; and so forth. Once people are aware that it is as appropriate to compliment as to criticize, they may be more likely actually to say those kind words, instead of leaving them unspoken and unheard.

College professors with large lecture classes rarely get any spontaneous feedback unless they are spectacularly good or horrible. The other 90 percent never really know what is getting across or how they are being received. And they never will unless they let their students know they need that feedback. They can do so in the form of anonymous evaluations or notes, which offset concerns about "buttering up" the grade-giver with flattery. Or the class can be encouraged to pass along the good and the "correctable flaws" to teaching assistants or class monitors. Whatever the mechanism, it should be part of the contract that governs the teaching relationship to exchange information about what can be done to improve one's performance and what deserves to be singled out for merit.

Positive experiences outside your primary area of work can also provide a needed balance to the negative and debilitating aspects of that work. In many cases, the experience that is most positive is contact with people who are healthy, happy, and free of major problems. Being with people for whom life is going well can be an important antidote to the negative bias arising from being with people for whom life is going badly.

> For example, one police officer in Tulsa photographs weddings in his spare time. Not only are these joyous occasions, but the people there are happy to see him—a situation quite different from his everyday work.
>
> One of the staff in Anaheim's probation department, who works with juvenile delinquents, coaches a neighborhood basketball team one afternoon a week. "I really look forward to that afternoon because I need to see average, normal kids who aren't in trouble and who are doing just fine. I need to see that kids' lives aren't always messed up, and that kids can be great to be with—I need it because my job could easily make me feel otherwise."

Although both of these examples refer to activities outside of work, a similar strategy can be used on the job. For instance, people taking care of cancer patients may try to offset the inherent emotional strain by spending some of their working hours with other types of patients:

> The pediatric oncologist who spends a month as a camp doctor with healthy youngsters each summer, the psychologist or social worker who has a private practice involving physically healthy clients in addition to seeing cancer patients at the hospital, and the nurse who "moonlights" two nights a month in the newborn nursery at a local maternity hospital all demonstrate this strategy.[5]

KNOW THYSELF People who recognize their need for these counterbalancing coping strategies are people who are tuned in to their inner feelings. They are sensitive to their personal reactions and are willing to reflect on the underlying reasons for them. This ability to introspect and understand yourself is critical for coping with burnout. The first step in knowing what action to take is to know what you are feeling and why.

> Eileen M., a clinical psychologist in a California county hospital, began to realize that there were certain patients whom she did not like and with whom she did a poor job of therapy. These patients were all female and displayed a passive, overly dependent, "whining" style of behavior. By analyzing her reactions to this type of woman (which were related to childhood experiences and her own professional training), Eileen was able to understand why her work with these patients was so unpleasant and upsetting. To alleviate this difficulty, she found professional colleagues who were more successful in treating such patients and arranged to refer these women to them.

The fact that Eileen was prepared to deal with other people's psychological problems probably made her more aware of her own. Moreover, her training as a therapist had sensitized her to issues of countertransference. She knew that her emotional reactions to patients were an important factor in the therapeutic relationship, and she knew that she had to come to terms with these reactions to work effectively and to maintain her emotional well-being. Research has found that therapists like Eileen, who have been trained to recognize and deal with countertransference, are better able than other therapists to handle the emotional exhaustion of burnout.[6]

Even without formal training in countertransference issues, you can benefit from a careful consideration of your personal feelings. This self-analysis is often enhanced by expressing your feelings verbally—by writing them down in a diary, talking into a tape recorder, or (as we shall see in Chapter 7) talking to a supportive colleague or friend. Such techniques force you to articulate and give shape to what may be vague and confusing feelings at first. They also serve a cathartic function, allowing you to "blow off steam" and let out emotional energy. Several weeks or months later a retrospective reflection on what you said earlier may provide new insights into your inner state.

Self-understanding begins with self-observation. What am I feeling? When, where, and with whom? What am I doing in response to that feeling? Keeping a daily log of these observations is an effective way to discover patterns of emotional stress.

DAILY STRESS AND TENSION LOG[7]

Description of physical signs of stress	Time of day	Where? Doing what? With whom?	What thoughts or feelings did I have?	What did I do in response to the stress?
1.				
2.				
3.				
4.				
5.				

This log should be kept on a daily basis for the *entire* day (including time at home as well as at work). For example:

1. Headache, tight neck muscles, fatigue	2:30 P.M.	At work, doing intake with new clients	Frustration, anger	Took a coffee break

2. Tension, insomnia	11:00 P.M.	At home, trying to fall asleep	Thinking about mistakes I made, worrying about tomorrow	Watched TV, took a tranquilizer

Record this information for two weeks, and then examine it for patterns of emotional response, possible causes, and styles of coping. For example, you may find that feelings of anxiety arise whenever you are dealing with older people or authority figures. Or perhaps irritability seems to peak in the late morning hours, regardless of the situation. Armed with this information, you can begin to explore possible answers to the next questions: *Why* am I feeling this way? What could I do about it that would be better than what I am now doing? For instance, knowing that certain times of day are problematic, you can try to schedule more low-key tasks for those periods (and do the more emotionally stressful work at another time), or schedule a break at that point (instead of earlier or later), or do different activities during that break (such as leaving the building and taking a short walk instead of staying at your desk and drinking coffee), and so forth. Choose coping techniques that are tailored to fit your personal needs within a particular situation. Your informed choice can only be based on an informed understanding of yourself.

A note of caution: self-analysis should be constructive, not destructive. Tearing yourself apart for all your flaws and failures is not the same as recognizing your limitations and learning from your mistakes. The former is an example of the self-blame and self-victimization I discussed in Chapter 1. The latter is an important step in self-improvement and personal growth. In addition, acknowledging your strengths is as central to self-understanding as admitting your weaknesses.

REST AND RELAXATION When people experience chronic stress, they often display a set of physical symptoms including tense muscles (especially in the face and neck), increased blood pressure, and an upset stomach that feels "tied up in knots." Not only are these symptoms unpleasant, they have serious long-term implications for health. In particular, high blood pressure is a major cause of heart attacks and strokes. Reduction of these health risks can be achieved by learning how to relax, both physically and mentally. Indeed, relaxation techniques are often at the heart of various stress management programs. Since people who burn out often suffer from these same physical symptoms, learning to relax can be an effective way for them to cope with this type of chronic emotional stress.

Relaxation techniques come in many forms. One person may choose meditation, another may utilize a biofeedback procedure, and still another may opt for an imagery technique (like the ones presented in the Appendix). However, the key to their effectiveness is the same in all cases: Practice. It does not matter what you do so long as you actually *do* it. This means setting aside the necessary time every day and practicing the procedures until they become second nature to you (probably in a few weeks). Regular relaxation will yield a significant reduction in stress symptoms.

Most relaxation techniques can be practiced easily during regular breaks in your work routine—such as lunch breaks, coffee breaks, or (for parents or child-care workers) children's nap time. They can also be practiced just before some event that you know will be stressful, such as that important public speech or evaluation session. Although ten to fifteen minutes is often the ideal amount of time for these techniques, there are also "quick" versions (such as the Instant Relaxation Drill presented in the Appendix) that can be done within a minute or two. Their advantage is flexibility—they can be done almost anywhere at almost any time (sitting or standing, waiting in line, taking a breather between clients). A tape recorder in your car, purse, or briefcase makes it possible to listen to programmed relaxation tapes while commuting to or from work (which is usually just dead time). However, mastery of these short techniques requires prior mastery of the longer ones and, as always, regular practice is essential.

A word of warning: Symptoms of stress are signals of an overloaded system, and that message should not be ignored in the rush to relax. Treating the symptom is not the same as treating the cause, and elimination of the symptom should not delude people into thinking that the cause of the problem has also disappeared. Unfortunately, we have learned to handle stress just like TV ads tell us to handle pain—take the fastest acting pill to stop the symptoms. Pain that recurs is telling you that something is wrong; stress sends the same message.

> Several groups of nurses on the East Coast learned various relaxation techniques to cope with stress. However, a later follow-up found that the nurses making greatest use of these techniques were having the most problems. What had gone wrong? Apparently, the nurses who learned to relax were now interpreting their lack of stress symptoms as a sign that "I'm strong, I'm feeling fine, I can handle anything now" and so they were taking on more responsibilities and working harder than ever before. Instead of alleviating stress, this coping strategy exacerbated it.

The lesson to be learned here is to listen to what your body is telling you—pay heed to the warning, even if you get rid of the signal.

MAKING THE TRANSITION Bringing home the burnout can be hazardous to your home life. The tension and emotional strain of work are not easily left behind and can be bad for relationships with family and friends. To cope with this problem, you should think of work and home as two very different environments and recognize that a special transition is needed to get from one to the other. Let me illustrate by using the analogy of scuba diving. A diver who makes a very deep descent has moved into an environment of high atmospheric pressure. If the diver returns too quickly to the surface, with its normal atmospheric pressure, he or she will get the "bends" (a painful and even paralyzing condition caused by the release of nitrogen bubbles into the bloodstream). To avoid this, the diver must make a gradual transition out of the high-pressure environment and *decompress.* In a similar way, people working in an environment of high emotional pressure need to decompress—to get completely out of that high-pressure environment before moving into the "normal pressure" of their private life.

But just what is decompression for a provider, as opposed to a diver? As I have defined it, *decompression* refers to some activity that: (a) occurs between one's working and nonworking times, and (b) allows one to unwind, relax, and leave the job behind before getting fully involved with family and friends. The activity is often in sharp contrast to the typical work routine. Since the emphasis in caregiving occupations is usually on problem solving and intellectual skills, many decompression activities avoid mental exertion. Little or no original thinking is necessary, and thinking about the job is brought to a halt. On the other hand, since many of these jobs involve minimal physical exertion, exercise is often a key element in decompression. As you might expect, there are many different activities that could serve the purpose of decompression. From among this infinite variety, you might try several methods and choose those that work best for you.

Many decompression activities are solitary ones. After a period of emotional overload, it is natural to want to get away from people and their problems and to have some peace, quiet, and time for oneself. The individual who gains this restorative solitude through a decompression activity is less likely to do so by isolating him- or herself from loved ones. Whether the activity involves exercise or rest, is planned or spontaneous is probably less important than the fact that it gives the person some privacy and the chance to be self-indulgent.

> Some people reserve this time for reading books (whether they be great classics or trashy novels), while others use it for a particular hobby (developing pictures in a darkroom, for example). Some write letters to friends, some take a long walk or window shop, some sit and daydream, and still others find a place where they can close the door, lie down, and take a nap. People who commute can often use this time to decompress. For those who take a bus or train, there is an opportunity to read or rest. For those who drive a car, there is the chance to listen to music or a favorite sports event. Sharon A., a rehabilitation counselor, went one step farther in her constructive use of the commute. She installed a tape deck in her car and now plays language instruction cassettes to help herself learn Italian. In addition to being interesting and useful, this language practice provides a clear break from her job activities. Furthermore, the concentration that it requires forces Sharon to stop thinking about her work and rehashing the day's problems—and thus it helps her make a successful

transition from work to home. She can also plan more realistically for a vacation in Venice someday.

The importance of being alone does not negate the importance of being with others. As we shall see later, there are many coping techniques that depend on people's presence, rather than their absence—such as socializing with friends after work, talking things over with your spouse, or consulting with a co-worker. However, you must realize that *both* solitude and socializing are necessary for handling burnout, and that people need time away as well as time together. "There's just times people be's tired of people," an Atlanta clerk reminded me.

Whether done alone or with company, a favorite hobby or interest is an ideal candidate for a decompression activity. Many people read, some play music, and still others engage in some artistic activity (painting, photography, pottery). Carpentry, stamp collecting, gourmet cooking—these and many other leisure activities can be used as the vehicle for transition from work to home.

A sport or physical exercise is another highly effective way to decompress. Many choices are available, depending on your personal preference and physical fitness. You might jog around the park or walk around the neighborhood. You might work out in a gym or take a dance class. You might ride a bicycle or go roller-skating or take a swim. You might join friends in playing tennis, touch football, or basketball. (A word of caution: If you are a poor loser who will really suffer the agony of defeat, a competitive sport is *not* the way for you to relax.) Whatever the exercise, its advantages are many. It helps you break away from work by making you function in a completely different mode. It can have a cathartic effect, allowing you to work off tension that has accumulated during the day. It contributes to your overall health, making you stronger and more resilient to stress and illness. The experience of Ronald S., a vocational rehabilitation counselor specializing in psychiatric disabilities, provides testimony for the power of physical activity as a way to decompress:

> I think a large part of my ability to cope with burnout is that for years I have been a competing AAU weight lifter. The hobby is excellent diversion from the very complex, abstract, tension-producing work of vocationally rehabilitating chronic mental patients. The three-hour workout sessions allow me a chance to become totally concrete, physical, and at times even primitive. The opportunity to ventilate physically and actually concretely "build" myself has a tremendous prophylactic effect against burnout.

Physical tension can also be alleviated in less energetic ways. You can unwind and relax by soaking in a hot bath, sitting in a sauna, taking a nap, or getting a massage. This physical relaxation can promote mental relaxation as well.

> Jeff B. works with juvenile offenders in southern California. His decompression activity takes place at home, in the large hot tub that he built himself. "I spend at least a half hour in the tub. I turn on the Jacuzzi and just listen

> to the sound of the bubbles—and my attention is on that peaceful sound and not on the day's events. So pretty soon I have stopped thinking about what happened at work and have just tuned everything out. By the time I get out of the tub, I'm feeling really relaxed and refreshed, and I'm ready to be with my family. My kids can see what it does for me—the rule is, "talk to Daddy *after* he's been in the tub, not before."

Jeff's technique of concentrating on the bubbles parallels the method of focused attention in various forms of meditation. Another analagous procedure is used by Lori R., who is a staff member of a suicide prevention center in California. After leaving work she goes to a nearby park, sits next to the duck pond, and just watches the ducks for a while. "It may sound silly, but it *is* a very calm and peaceful thing to do—it's simple, it doesn't make demands on me, and I just don't bother to worry about anything else."

For many decompression activities the underlying theme is: "Slow down—you move too fast." No matter what you do, make the pace less hurried and less hectic than your regular work routine. Even when there is little time to be set aside for a special activity, you can still take it slow and easy. For example, rather than racing to catch the first bus, you might wait at the bus stop and let a few go by. Or take a few minutes just to sit and relax in your car before going home. Although they may not sound like much, such calculated slowdowns help put the brakes on the daily rat race.

A LIFE OF ONE'S OWN What do you do when you are not at work? What are you besides your job title? If you have a lot of answers to these questions, then you have an effective strategy for handling burnout. There is more to your life than your work, and that "more" can offset the emotional strain of that work and help you "recharge your batteries." However, it is a sign of trouble if your nonworking hours are just that—an *absence* of work, rather than a *presence* of something else. When your whole world is your work and little else, then your whole world is more likely to fall apart when problems arise on the job. Your sense of competence, your self-esteem, and your personal identity are all based on what you do in life, and they will be far more shaky and insecure if that base is a narrow one. The lesson to be learned here is the importance of a rich and varied private life to complement the public one. Or, to rephrase Irving Berlin, do *not* put all of your eggs in one basket.

The first step in strengthening your private life is to protect it from encroachments by your work. Setting up clear boundaries between job and home means that when you leave the job, you really *leave* it—psychologically as well as physically.

> As one psychiatric nurse put it during an interview, "If you let things upset you a lot, then you can't enjoy any time that you are away from the ward. I mean, what I do, my job—I enjoy it very much, and I do it eight

hours a day, and I do it the best I can. But when I go home, that's it. I'm gone, and the ward is here, and I'm home."

But keeping your job out of your home life is easier said than done. Pieces of your private time get taken over by your job every time you: (1) rehash the day's problems at home, (b) take home work to do in the evening or on weekends, (c) work overtime, or (d) are "on call." How do you handle this? In many cases, the solution is to say *no.* No to too much overtime, no to daily homework, no to continuous "on call." Saying no does not mean saying never; extra work may be essential at times or may be required by your job. However, saying no can put limits on these extras–for example, "I'll arrange to be on call only three nights a week." "I will not bring work home on Tuesdays because that is going to be my regular bowling night." "No matter what comes up, Saturdays are reserved for my family." Or (in the case of mothers whose work *is* family) "one afternoon a week I get a baby-sitter and get out of the house for some time to myself." Sticking to these limits can be difficult, because your work will always make increasing demands of you ("Well, I'll do it just this once"; "They really need me, so what else can I do?" "It's an emergency"). So enlist your family or friends as enforcers ("Hey, no cheating, Dad–it's Saturday") to prevent you from backsliding.

Bringing home the emotional turmoil of the job is perhaps the most insidious way to let your work overrun your private life. It is hard to put a stop to recurring thoughts and unresolved feelings and to avoid venting them on the nearest target. Decompression activities help deal with this problem. Another technique is a cooling-off period of an hour or so once you are at home. During this time the rule is, "nothing negative." Whatever you talk about with your friends, spouse, or kids, it has to be something pleasant–such as an interesting TV program, vacation plans, or a funny incident at work. Gripes and complaints are strictly forbidden.

Two things happen as a result of a cooling-off period. First, you ensure a pleasant time with the people you care about most. Second, your problems become less immediate and less intense–and perhaps less important, as you gain some distance from them. If you then talk about these problems later on with your spouse or friend, you will probably be able to do so in a more calm and constructive way.

Having set aside some private time, the next step is to *do* something with it. Leisure activities of any kind are a great help in handling burnout. Not only are these "mini-vacations" a diversion from job tensions, but they can provide positive experiences with other people and can give an important boost to your sense of competence and self-esteem. They replenish and rejuvenate and thus offset the exhaustion and emptiness of burnout. By giving *to* yourself you will feel more able to give *of* yourself to others.

Leisure activities can take many forms. Hobbies, sports, art, music, and literature are all valuable pursuits during your private time, as are entertainment and travel. Choose whatever is most fun and rewarding for you, but be sure to translate those choices into *action.* Good intentions are not good ways to cope.

In some cases, a leisure activity may become an avocation or even a second job. Moonlighting is often done to earn extra income or develop new job skills, but it is also an effective coping technique. If moonlighting brings you into contact with individuals under pleasant and rewarding circumstances, then it can offset the negative reaction toward people that is so characteristic of burnout. Some examples that I gave earlier were the cancer caregivers who "moonlighted" with healthy children, the police officer who worked occasionally as a wedding photographer, and the teacher who was a lifeguard during the summer.

Although privacy and solitude are a part of one's private life, many "off hours" are spent in the company of others. These other people–whether they be family, friends, or acquaintances–are important allies in your battle against burnout. They are a source of aid and comfort, of recognition and rewards, of good feelings and pleasurable experiences. A recurrent finding in my research is the importance of a good marriage or intimate relationship in handling burnout. The emotional support it provides is a counterbalance to the emotional drain of the job. Successes in one's personal relationships can be an effective antidote to feelings of frustration or failure in one's professional contacts. "I could not ease my client's troubles today, but I did make my spouse feel happy (or friend, neighbor, child, parent)." Personal strength often comes from strong social supports. Research shows that people who are part of a solid social support network are better able to cope with physical ills and psychological problems.[8]

Personal strength can also come from a strong religious faith or spiritual philosophy. These beliefs can give meaning to work, provide hope and inspiration in adversity, and be a source of comfort and joy in an otherwise bleak institution. People in religious callings often say their relationship with God is what led them to that line of work and what keeps them going when the duties are difficult or require self-sacrifice. But you do not need to be a church-affiliated religious professional to gain such benefits.

> A group of police officers in San Francisco (nicknamed Cops for Christ, or the God Squad) use their religious faith to cope with the stress of their work and to minimize its negative personal consequences (such as alcoholism, family problems). During weekly meetings they pray, discuss the Bible and use it to help them deal with the aftermath of crime. Said one officer, "The pressures, the hours of police work, of seeing people at their worst, it's bound to have an effect on you. If you don't understand the nature of evil, if you don't understand why, then you can start believing that everything is evil." For another officer, a thirty-year veteran of the streets, faith has played an important part in his emotional well-being. "I'm just as tough as I ever was. But now I've learned compassion, learned that tenderness has to go along with toughness if you're going to accomplish anything. I used to be hard, indifferent, but not anymore. I've surrendered my heart to Jesus."[9]

CHANGING JOBS If, in spite of all your best efforts, the job situation has not improved, you may realize that it is time for you to go. Giving up a job is a serious step to take, and a decision to do so should be based on careful consideration of the underlying reasons and available alternatives. Quitting can be costly, both financially and psychologically. Nevertheless, the best solution may be a permanent leave rather than a temporary one.

For some people, changing jobs may mean a change within their profession. A different organization or position might be involved, as when a teacher shifts to a new school or teaches a different grade level. A word of caution, however: If the change is more superficial than real, then the risk of burnout is not really reduced. Going into the same type of job situation and handling it in the same way as before does not represent progress. More major job changes include moving into administrative work or training rather than direct care. Here the changes in the content and context of the job are usually more substantial. However, for some people, changing jobs means the more extreme decision to leave the profession entirely. A Chicago schoolteacher who now runs a physical fitness salon is one example.

Finally, it is important to realize that while many changes are for the better, some changes are not. Change does not automatically guarantee success and happiness. Make your expectations realistic ones and be prepared for mistakes. Nevertheless, well-planned change can be a positive step in personal growth and should be considered crucial to the process of taking stock of yourself in order to take better care of yourself.

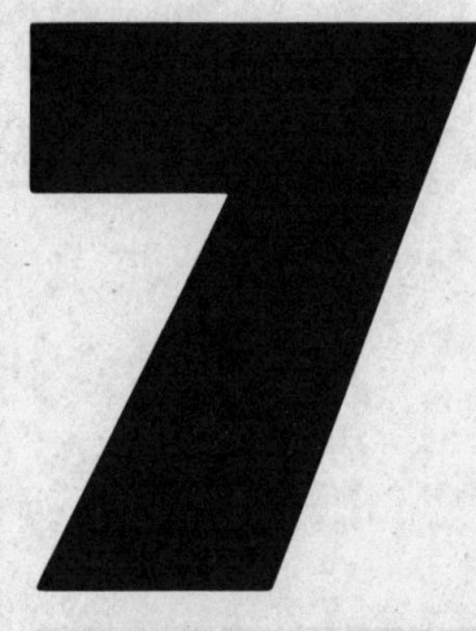

HOW TO HANDLE BURNOUT: SOCIAL AND ORGANIZATIONAL APPROACHES

My colleagues and I get together periodically, and that helps us deal with a problem. We bitch a lot to each other. We hash things out. We laugh at it sometimes. We talk about it a lot and try new ways. It helps to talk about it, and if you can't see it another way, then somebody else might be able to. There are some clients that everybody feels are incredibly hard to work with, so then we put our heads together to come up with a new solution. Sometimes we even go outside and get some kind of consultant.

Charles T., social worker

Working overly long hours is really the first sign of burnout. Nurses start working ten, twelve hours a day, four and five days a week, saying they can't go home because there's too much to do. One of my responsibilities is to watch for this sign, and if I find people continually staying ten hours instead of eight, then I talk to them about it. I remind them that we have three shifts for a very good reason, and I suggest they go home and let the next shift take over. This happens to head nurses and supervisors, too. When it does, we sit down and discuss what they're feeling, what they can do about it, what kind of help they need with their job. A lot of times I tell them to take four days off and relax.[1]

You can do a lot on your own to deal with burnout, but you can do even more with a little help from your friends (and colleagues, supervisors, boss, and others). They can be your aides and allies, rather than your adversaries. They can be a source of strength and support, rather than an additional drain on your time and energy. As we saw in Chapter 3, your place of work and the people with whom you work can be negative factors in burnout. However, as we shall see here, they also have a more positive potential to prevent burnout.

SOCIAL SUPPORT

Getting away from people is a common response when emotional overload is high. The desire for peace and privacy is certainly understandable, and these needs can be satisfied in constructive ways. However, occasional solitude is not the same as frequent isolation. The drawback comes when getting away from others is overdone to the point where you cut yourself off from some valuable resources. Getting together with people is just as important (if not more so) than getting away from them. People can provide many things that you cannot provide for yourself–new information and insights, training in new skills, recognition and feedback, emotional support, advice, and help of various kinds. Some of these things can be provided by a spouse or close friend. But in many cases, the people who are best qualified to provide job-related help and support are the people on the job–your co-workers.

The Companionship of Colleagues

The power of your peers to help you handle burnout should not be underestimated. Indeed, they can be your most valuable resource. You can get support from your fellow workers through formal or official mechanisms, such as professional support groups or staff meetings. However, informal get-togethers are more common–such as talking with co-workers over lunch or during breaks or socializing with them after working hours. Whatever the format, the social and emotional support provided by peers can be critical for survival on the job. An example is the teaching profession:

> It has become clear, especially in teaching the emotionally disturbed, that a teacher can not function adequately for long without an informed shoulder to lean on, without an on-the-spot human wailing wall at which to gripe, to rage, to express fears and confess mistakes, to ask questions and wonder aloud . . . where the human wailing wall is carefully conceived and consistently offered, where the people provided are . . . informed, sensitive, sympathetic, and understanding, the turnover among teachers, even under the most incredibly difficult conditions, is remarkably lowered.[2]

How do peers help you with burnout? Basically, they reduce the emotional strain, either by doing something about the source of stress or by getting you to cope with it more effectively.

HELP Doing something about the source of stress is when your peers get you out of a tough situation. They might give you some direct aid (such as coming to your assistance when a client gets particularly rude or threatening) or teach you how to handle a certain problem. They might take over your duties temporarily, allowing you to withdraw from an upsetting situation.

> For example, one psychiatric nurse told me about the emotional strain of working with a particular suicidal patient.
>
> "She had done some very bizarre kinds of things to herself—cutting her Achilles tendon, slitting her throat in a very gross way, slitting her wrists. She set herself on fire several times on the ward. I spent an eight-hour shift working with her, and I was so down by the time I left that I knew I couldn't keep doing this. I talked to the other staff about it and made my needs known to them. So then, whenever I had worked a few hours with this woman and it was really beginning to get to me, another staff member would work with her or get her included in some group activity. Meanwhile, I would take a breather and try to get back on top of the situation. And I do the same sort of things for the other staff because they have patients that they're working with that they don't want to spend eight hours with either."

COMFORT Stress reduction also takes the form of comfort and emotional support. Peers can provide a shoulder to cry on and a sympathetic ear—"I know what you're going through, I understand how you feel, I've been there myself." It is easier to express your thoughts and feelings to a friendly audience—in this case, people who are familiar with the situation and who have a similar status and perspective on it. As one nurse put it: "There is no time or opportunity to say how you really feel when you are continually under the eye of doctors, nursing assistants, supervisors, patients, and patients' families. What nurses need most is other nurses to hear their problems and help them find more rewards in what they do."

INSIGHT Peers can help you out of a rut by giving you a new perspective on the problem. They can help you see things differently (as Charles T. pointed out in the opening statement). They may be able to express the thoughts and feelings that you find uncomfortable to say yourself. And they can help you analyze your own feelings and gain some insight into your reactions. A good example of this is provided by Erin C., a psychiatric nurse in California:

> Sometimes I get really angry with patients. At that point, it helps to talk with another nurse to figure out *why* I'm angry. Is it my own limitation, my own lack of experience, or is it because of their pathology that I can't

get through to them, that nobody can get through to them, or is it that I'm just irritable that day and I'm not good to discuss much of anything with anybody?

COMPARISON Peers also provide you with a basis for personal comparison. Their feelings and actions can serve as a yardstick against which to measure your own. This comparison function is particularly useful when you are unsure of how appropriate or how typical your reactions are. "Is it normal to feel this way? Am I overreacting? Am I the only one who feels like this?" By talking to your colleagues you will usually discover that you are *not* alone and that your feelings are indeed shared by others. Such comparative knowledge can help correct the bias toward self-blame that I discussed in Chapter 1.

> A vivid example of the need for personal comparison is the reactions of emergency personnel in the 1978 air crash in San Diego, which I mentioned in Chapter 3. The extent of human carnage and chaos made the rescue and clean-up work especially traumatic, and the workers' emotional feelings were often overwhelming. About one hundred of them sought therapeutic help, and their most immediate need was for knowledge that they were normal. They needed to find out that they were not weak or crazy to have reacted so strongly, and that anyone else would have reacted in the same way to that situation. Indeed, many of them urged their therapists to view films and pictures of the crash site—partly as a way of convincing the therapists (and themselves) that their reactions were justified by the extreme horror of the situation.

Emotional comparison is essential when we are uncertain about what we are feeling but know that the arousal is negative. Often anxieties come without labels, are disruptive, and seem inappropriate to the current situation. "There is no rational reason for me to be upset at this time." But, in fact, there may be many good reasons of which you are not consciously aware. Your coping reaction to a threat may have suppressed the anxiety about your vulnerability, which surfaces later when you are not in a danger situation requiring action. Or this nice client may resemble another whom you disliked. Maybe some anxiety at home (such as the suspicion that your spouse is losing affection for you) is being carried over into the job. Whatever the true cause, it is by comparing your emotional reaction to others in the same situation that you can evaluate better whether it is a reaction to some subtle, unrecognized aspect of the work setting (if others share the reaction), or if it is an idiosyncrasy—something you are bringing into the job setting. If it is the latter, and it persists, psychological counseling may be in order.

REWARDS Not only can peers tell you if you are socially and emotionally normal, they can tell you if you are good. The most important (and perhaps only) source of praise, compliments, and recognition for a job well done may be your fellow workers. Not only are they in a good position to evaluate what you've done, but they may be in the best position to give you feedback that is both immediate and meaningful. Praise from a peer often has greater impact and is more highly treasured than a general performance rating and gold star from one's superiors. To get positive feedback, you may have to ask for it—just as you do with recipients.

However, the best tactic for getting feedback is first to *give* positive feedback to others. The golden rule of "doing unto others as you would have them do unto you" is especially true here. While you are waiting for a co-worker to compliment your work, remember that *you* are the colleague that someone else is hoping to hear from. Take the first step of rewarding others for their accomplishments—notice all the things they do well and tell them so.

HUMOR Humor is another important coping technique that requires the presence of peers. Jokes and laughter can reduce emotional strain by making things seem less serious, less frightening, and less overwhelming. The battlefield surgeons in "M*A*S*H," who joke and flirt with the nurses while performing grave operations, are a particularly good example of this technique at work. Moreover, humor injects a positive element into what may otherwise be a bleak situation, lifting everyone's spirits. A good illustration of humor in action comes from the staff of one cancer unit, who "spontaneously organized a kazoo band and marched from room to room playing request numbers for the patients."[3] Making jokes may be hard in some situations (as when a patient is dying), but just those situations may be where laughter is needed most and is, indeed, "the best medicine."

> Mr. Z., who was dying of lung cancer, had requested that he spend his last days at home instead of in the hospital. Ms. C. was one of the private nurses who was assisting his family in taking care of him. She not only joked with Mr. Z., but some of her jokes had a sexual innuendo, as in "Oh, Mr. Z., now that's not what I meant when I asked if you were getting up!" Although some people regarded such jokes as inappropriate, they actually did a lot of good for both the nurse and her patient. She was able to brighten a grim situation and know that she was making someone's final hours more pleasant. And Mr. Z. was able to feel that his lively "old self" was still there, a welcome ally in the face of impending death.

Humor can be helpful, but it is important to recognize that it has its harmful side as well. If you begin to laugh *at* people, instead of laughing with them, then humor becomes cruel. Humor that puts people down only adds to the callousness of burnout and becomes a means by which derogatory feelings are expressed. I have found the relationship of negative humor to burnout in my studies with such diverse groups as police and health care professionals. Laughing at the expense of others is often done to protect oneself, as one nurse explained:

> Sometimes things are so frustrating that to keep from crying, you laugh at a situation that may not be funny. You laugh, but you know in your heart

what's really happening. Nevertheless, you do it because your own needs are important—we're all human beings and we have to be ourselves."

Although negative humor may serve some personal needs, it is very costly in terms of the needs of others, especially their need for respect. Thus, the use of humor must be exercised with care, to maximize its healthy effects and minimize its hazardous ones.

ESCAPE In addition to helping you see the bright (or funny) side of things, your peers can also help take you away from it all. Temporary escapes from the rigors of work can be done on your own, but doing them with others may be more effective. You can "get away" from work more completely during your breaks by talking with your co-workers about the latest movie, your vacation plans, or the weekend football game than you can just by thinking about these topics. Your colleagues can get you involved in something else, for a short period, and ensure a real change of pace in your regular routine.

Keep in mind, however, that it is just as possible to overdo your involvement with colleagues as it is to overdo isolating yourself from them. There is always the danger of the "wartime romance"—an attraction to a co-worker as a way of escaping the pressures or tedium of the job, rather than because of that individual's inherent qualities. The question to ask is, "Would I still be so attracted to this person if I were in an ideal situation?" If the answer is "probably not" or "I'm not so sure," then you should realize that your relationship is serving a purpose other than love and friendship. Heavy involvement with your colleagues, to the exclusion of other relationships, should be viewed as a warning sign rather than as a functional coping strategy.

Getting It Together

It is one thing to say how helpful colleagues can be, but quite another to get that potential help translated into reality. In jobs where the provider is relatively isolated, the difficulty in just getting access to peer support can be a major problem.

> During my interviews with several psychiatrists, some of them reported being part of a social-professional support group when they were doing their residency. They would meet regularly to discuss problems that they were having in treating their patients, to vent frustrations, or to report their successes. After leaving the hospital and entering private practice, some of these psychiatrists found that the lack of such a group was a serious, unanticipated loss to them. "I felt cut off, isolated—I didn't feel I had people to whom I could turn when problems arose and whose opinions I could trust," one therapist told me. Some psychiatrists even made efforts to rejoin the hospital meetings of the residents, although not always successfully.

A similar sort of isolation from peers can occur for mothers who are alone in their homes with their kids and who do not have an extended family (parents, grandparents, aunts) living nearby. Developing contacts with other mothers (through parent-participation nursery schools, neighborhood car pools, or the proverbial morning *kaffeeklatsch*) can be the route to gaining peer support.

Getting in touch with your colleagues, then, is an important first step—whether it be at staff meetings, during lunch breaks, after working hours, at parties, or at staff development activities (such as conferences or retreats). But after the initial contact, then what? The next step is to determine what group mechanism can provide the basis for peer support. In many cases, such a group already exists in the form of work teams, a work partner (or "buddy system"), or friendship groups. In other cases, a new group needs to be established. This can be done on a formal basis, setting up a regular meeting to deal specifically with staff issues, or informally, as when some people decide to talk things over during the Thursday lunch hour.

No matter what type of group is set up, the key element is *trust.* People should feel comfortable with each other and have faith that they all have one another's best interests at heart. Such trust is essential if people are going to reveal their feelings, problems, and possibly their own shortcomings in an effort to gain aid and comfort. A certain vulnerability is involved in being open with others, and if someone thinks that those others will exploit rather than respect it, that person is likely to close up rather than open up. If group members are competing with each other (for promotions, attention, status) or if rivalries, one-upmanship tactics, or strong feelings of dislike are present, then the group is in *no* shape to serve as a source of social support. Other groups that *are* characterized by mutual trust should be sought out for this purpose. Or, if the group is a newly formed one, considerable time and effort should be spent on first establishing a sense of trust and cooperation before getting involved in other activities.

A support group usually works best if it has some sort of leader. This is the person who keeps the group on track—who makes sure that problems are being aired and dealt with, that feedback is constructive, that personal hassles or disputes are ironed out, and that everybody has a chance to say what's on his or her mind. A good leader is often the key difference between an effective support group and an ineffective (or even counterproductive) one. While some leaders are just "naturals," more often a good leader is someone who is well trained in these necessary skills. This is especially true when the group has been formally organized as part of a stress reduction program and needs someone to provide direction and structure. For example, in New York City's Beth Israel Hospital, the stress groups for nurses are run by a psychiatrist. In other places the group leader might be a psychologist, or a social worker, or someone else with special training in directing groups.

Open and honest communication is more likely to occur among co-workers if supervisory staff are not present. People will be more frank if they feel they are among friends and not under the watchful eye of a boss. When supervisors or administrators are part of the group, people will be guarded in their behavior because they are worried about evaluations and future job consequences. In arguing for groups of peers, I am not dismissing the importance of get-togethers between supervisors and staff. As we shall see later, meetings between different levels of personnel can be critical for resolving conflicts and disagreements. However, the various support and helping functions I have discussed so far are best provided by colleagues.

The Role of Group Ritual

Think back to the example in the last chapter of Jeff B. sitting in his hot tub. Did you react a little negatively to that image of self-indulgence? I know I did when I first heard it. But now consider that in Japan it is assumed that most businessmen will go regularly to the hot baths after work with a small group of their colleagues. There they relax physically and socialize before heading to their homes. Because this stop has become a ritual practice within the group and the society, individuals are exempt from being thought to be overindulging themselves. One important role of organized rituals is the permission they grant individuals to participate in certain actions without having to justify them in terms of personal motivations or excuse them as necessary to achieve some personal goal. When everyone does it, people can allow themselves to go with the ritualized flow of the group and not be held accountable as individuals for doing what they believe is in their best interests but might not have the courage or resources to do on their own.

Potential Pitfalls

One of the primary hazards of any group get-together is the bitch session. When people gather to talk about their troubles, there is an almost overwhelming tendency for all to pitch in with their own personal sob stories—"Let me tell you how bad it is for *me*"; "If you think *that's* bad, wait until you hear this"; and so forth. Undoubtedly, this "ain't-it-awful" bitch session is motivated by a need to get things off the chest. But catharsis alone is not a very constructive way to cope. Releasing pent-up feelings may feel good at first, but if it is not followed by new insights into how to do things better, it is not particularly helpful. Furthermore, if you think you are depressed or upset by your own problem, imagine how you will feel after hearing ten more of them! So beware of the bitch session—it is an unproductive and even destructive "downer" for everyone concerned.

A second hazard for support groups is the confrontation session. For those who are already emotionally exhausted, an encounter session in which people begin to challenge, criticize, and even attack each other can be extremely debilitating. Even when the expressed purpose of such sessions is honest communication and personal growth, an emotionally demanding encounter may not be the best means of reaching that goal, especially for helpers who are already emotionally overwrought. According to one therapist who has dealt extensively with burnout in free clinic settings:

> The encounter group experience is tremendously draining on the emotions, and would be especially so to one who has burnt out. What he needs at this point is understanding, comfort, support and building up—and love. What he definitely does not need is to be torn down.[4]

Resistance to group participation is a third potential problem area. Some people may be reluctant to get together with others, for various reasons. They may assume that group meetings will be encounter group sessions—which they want no part of. They may believe that group meetings are just a waste of their valuable time and an ineffective way to cope with stress. They may be "loners" who feel uncomfortable in social situations or who would prefer to do things on their own. Whatever the underlying reason for their reluctance, it should be respected. Imposing "groupiness" on an unwilling participant is not going to win any converts to the cause. However, developing a group that *is* an effective source of support and making such an alternative available to people may be the best way to stimulate more contact among colleagues.

IMPROVEMENTS IN THE WORK PLACE

Burnout is fostered by certain types of work environments. The nature of the job—what people have to do, and when and where they do it—are often the source of the chronic emotional stresses they struggle to cope with. But people can do more than just cope with the environment—they can try to change it. Making modifications and instituting improvements in the work setting are indeed within the realm of possibility (contrary to the often-expressed skepticism that organizations are too big and too set in their ways to change). Admittedly, it is always easier to stick with the status quo and to keep on doing things in the old familiar way. However, when the status quo gets costly (in terms of turnover, absenteeism, poor performance), most organizations will be receptive to new ideas. New ideas may come from within, suggested by staff or management, but they can also come from outside consultants, particularly when workers are too close to the problem to see obvious avenues of change.

There are several reasons why it is important to push for organizational changes, and not just personal ones. First, although individual coping techniques may be quicker and easier, improvements of the work place may have a more pervasive and long-lasting impact on rates of burnout. Teaching people how to cope with a stressful job is certainly helpful, but it may not be as effective as making the job less stressful to begin with. Second, organizational changes acknowledge the significance of the situation in burnout. This can counter the overwhelming (and somewhat erroneous) tendency to blame either oneself or one's recipients. Third, an organizational response to burnout constitutes recognition of it as a legitimate problem. For many years the problem of burnout was either pooh-poohed or swept under the rug. It was not acceptable to talk about it or to request special considerations because of it. Once organizations recognize that burnout *is* a real and serious problem for them and their employees, then greater efforts may be made to deal effectively with it.

> Several years ago, I had an interview with Randy L., a psychiatrist in the psychological services unit of a large medical organization. "If you react emotionally or get upset by certain highly stressful events or crises, it is considered understandable and legitimate to feel that way. For example, suppose there was a death in your family. People would be extremely sympathetic and supportive, and would try to help you out, would be tolerant of any slipups, and would even encourage you to get away for awhile. It would be OK for you to be feeling bad and OK for you to ask for help. But with burnout, it's not OK. I guess the "crisis" is not considered big enough or important enough—probably because it is not an emergency but is there all the time."

The sort of organizational changes I will be discussing here are not things you do on your own, as a single individual. Because they involve organizational policy, they require the combined efforts of people at various levels. The impetus for change might be staff complaints, or supervisors' reports, or administrators' worries, but the actual planning and successful implementation of change rests on the participation of all. The form of this participation will vary widely from one organization to another, depending on the size and structure of the organization, its bureaucracy and existing policies, its style of management, and so forth. Although the way organizational decisions are made and carried out is an important and relevant issue, I will not be discussing it here. Rather, I want to focus on the *types* of decisions that could be made with respect to burnout and show how these proposed changes might alleviate the problem.

A final caveat: Very few, if any, of these proposed changes have actually been tested to determine how truly effective they are. The reason for this lack of testing is not a lack of interest in finding out what works best. Rather, it is because the proper evaluation is extremely difficult to do—it is costly, it is time consuming, and it requires extensive cooperation from the participating organizations and their employees (which is not always readily forthcoming). The need for more of these evaluations is great. Without them, our knowledge of effective changes is limited, and our recommendations remain best guesses rather than established fact.

Getting More Resources

One of the most popular proposals for any type of problem (including burnout) is "more"—more staff, more money, more time, more facilities, more equipment. It is indeed true that more of these resources would alleviate some of the pressures that produce burnout. Heavy case loads could be reduced, people would not have to be "processed," successful achievements would be more likely, and so forth. If it is possible to get "more," then getting more should be given high priority.

But the possibility of getting more resources in these times of tight money is highly unlikely. While "more" may be the ideal, "less" is often the reality. At a time when funds are being cut back or even eliminated, the problem becomes how to get by on less, not how to get more. Thus, the more practical approach to burnout may be to find out what can be done differently and better regardless of available resources, rather than because of them.

Doing It Better

In Chapter 6 we saw how an individual could cope with stress by doing the same things differently. This advice holds true for organizations as well. A better division of labor, a rearrangement of job assignments, a change in standard operating procedure—all of these can go a long way toward reducing the risk of burnout.

DIVIDING UP THE WORK Within many organizations work is divided according to major job tasks. Task A is done by one person, Task B is done by someone else (who never does Task A), and so on. For example, one person deals directly with the public, while someone else handles administrative work. Contrast this with a system in which each person does several job tasks instead of a single one. Everyone has some contact with the public, but also at times everyone helps take care of administrative chores. In this way the same work has been divided differently.

What are the advantages of this different division? First, it makes the job more varied and interesting. An individual is not stuck in the boring routine of doing the same thing over and over again and is also acquiring a wider range of skills. An interesting job is not necessarily a less stressful one, but people will be more willing to stick with an interesting job and to try to find solutions for its problems.

A second advantage of this redivision is more directly related to burnout. Work that is emotionally draining can be counterbalanced by work that is not. People can handle the tough parts of a job better if they know that they can ease up later on.

For instance, working with dying patients is very emotionally demanding. In some institutions, caregivers are required to put limits on their direct

> service time to these patients and to spend some of their working hours doing very different tasks. They might spend a portion of their time doing teaching, or carrying out a research project, or handling administrative work.

This shift between more and less emotionally stressful tasks is the same principle underlying the coping technique of downshifts. However, with work variety this principle is made a regular part of the everyday routine, rather than being used only on stressful occasions by resourceful individuals. Furthermore, this sort of system is a more flexible one. If someone wants to pull out of one task because things are getting too tough, it is easier to find a replacement. And the person who pulls out can still be productive by doing some other needed work.

Dividing the work differently could also have another benefit. People who move up into administrative positions often have to leave behind the opportunity to work in direct service. They cannot return to this kind of work, even if they would like to do it some of the time, without suffering a loss in pay and prestige. A redivision of work responsibilities might be an effective solution.

> Joe B., a school district administrator in southern California, told me how much he missed teaching. "I liked working with kids–it was a very challenging job and I think I was pretty good at it. But how can I go back? It would be a real step down, given the system we have, and it would mean giving up my current job, which I also like. So I guess I'm stuck up here. But I would love to teach sometimes–maybe just a class here and there, nothing full-time–just to keep my hand in and not lose that contact with the kids."

What Joe B. wanted was this kind of work redivision–he wanted to do *both* administrative work and teaching, not one or the other. This idea sounds good in theory, but it may not always be practical. Dividing up certain job duties between several people may cause confusion and conflict and result in a lot of waste and inefficiency. However, the same goal can be achieved in another way–job rotation. Instead of doing several things simultaneously, people do them sequentially. For example, in the case of Joe B., he would spend a period of time in administration, then he would rotate into teaching for awhile, then he would rotate back into administration, and so forth. Job rotations, lateral job transfers, or cross-training can achieve many of the same effects as varied job tasks. They counterbalance one type of work with another. They can prevent people from getting into a rut and feeling trapped in their work. And they can renew and restore interest and energy.

> The restorative function of rotation is seen in the account of a therapist in an alternative self-help institution. "I recall one instance in which a woman who was an excellent clinician and encounter master had burned out. We put her in charge of purchasing food and clothing for the therapeutic community, a task that demanded no clinical confrontations, just a lot of talk

with suppliers, grocers, keeping track of goods, not people. She loved it. The shift helped us to save her both for herself and for us."[5]

Moving people between jobs may be easier to do than splitting the jobs between people, but it has its limitations as well. It will be an inefficient procedure if each rotation requires a great deal of training or a long "warm-up" time before staff people are handling things smoothly. It will be counterproductive if the rotations are done so frequently that staff do not have time to complete projects or get to know clients or patients very well. In the latter instance, it may even foster the unfeeling and uncaring depersonalization of burnout, since staff may feel less personally accountable to the people they serve.

CHANGING THE CONTACT WITH CLIENTS Involvement with people and their problems is a major source of emotional exhaustion. And these encounters with others can be made even more stressful by organizational regulations. So what is the obvious solution? Make some modifications in the operating procedure so that direct contact is less demanding. These modifications do not always have to be major policy changes that require an official seal of approval. They can be more minor and informal changes as well.

Two steps should be followed in developing such changes: (a) identify aspects of the client contact that can cause emotional strain, and (b) devise ways to alter those aspects. Obviously, if a change is to be successful, it has to be tailored to the specific needs and characteristics of the organization. For that reason, it will be impossible for me to make recommendations that would apply in all cases. Rather, I will give some examples of possible changes in the hope that they will at least stimulate other ideas if they are not used themselves.

The first example deals with clients' access to staff. Staff who are continuously "on call" and available to clients are more at risk for burnout. One modification of this availability policy would be to put limits on it. Instead of having everyone ready at all times, different people could be ready at different times. In other words, staff availability can be structured so that there is less unpredictability about client contact.

> In a day-care center that I studied with Ayala Pines, the prevailing philosophy had been one of nondirected permissiveness and openness. Staff had to be available at any time to anyone who came their way—whether children, parents, co-workers, or administrators. Schedules were irregular and activities unplanned and spontaneous, since no one could predict who would be around at any one time. Consequently, emotional exhaustion among the staff was high. To deal with this problem, the staff changed the policy of total availability. Each staff member was assigned a specific group of children for a specific time period. This structure allowed the staff member to establish better relationships with the children for whom he or she was responsible and to carry out a program that was planned and predictable instead of chaotic. Availability for some was better than availability for all—both for the staff and for the children.[6]

Getting and giving information is another potential problem area in staff-client relationships. This is especially true when the client feels embarrassed, ashamed, guilty, or afraid about revealing this knowledge to someone else. In these situations staff people have to be "nosy," and possibly even rude, as they probe for critical information. One alternative approach is to figure out a way to get the client to present the information voluntarily, so that the staff person does not have to ask a potentially awkward question ("Pardon me, but . . .").

> For example, dental X-rays are hazardous during the first few months of a woman's pregnancy, since the developing fetus is particularly vulnerable at that time. However, it is almost impossible to tell that a woman is in the early stage of pregnancy because she has not yet begun to "show." And the question, "Pardon me, but are you pregnant?" may be viewed as insulting or embarrassing by the woman who is not, since it may imply that she is getting fat. A better procedure would be to post a sign on the waiting-room door that says that being pregnant is an important bit of information for the dentist, and to please let him or her know about it. By cuing the patients in this way, the dental staff would not have to worry about "is she or isn't she?" and how to know for sure.

Getting and giving the same information over and over again can get tedious and boring. It can even be irritating to keep making the same arguments and handling the same objections repeatedly. When irritation infects the staff-client relationship, it breeds even more ill will and increases the stressfulness of the contact. Reducing redundancy is one way to break this escalation of emotional strain. Rather than going through the same process for each individual client, the staff member might devise "shortcut" procedures in which clients can be dealt with in groups. This is particularly useful when some basic information or orientation procedure is necessary for all clients before individual treatment. A single presentation at a group session can be just as effective (if not more so) than several presentations at each of several individual sessions. And it usually involves less time, less effort, and less emotional wear and tear.

Another source of strain in staff-client contacts is a mismatch in goals and expectations. This can be particularly problematic because the differing expectations are rarely expressed. The general approach to take here is to make things explicit. A procedure in which both clients and staff state their expectations can allow mismatches to be recognized and misunderstandings to be resolved. The limits of the staff-client relationship can be clarified, and, in some cases, the terms of this "contract" can be renegotiated. Clarifying expectations usually requires direct communication between client and staff. However, some of it can also be done with written forms (such as preliminary information sheets on what can and cannot be done by the staff members).

The passive-dependent stance of many clients can be another emotional burden for staff. Staff can deal with this by devising ways of giving clients more independence and responsibility for taking care of themselves, thus alleviating some of the demands placed on them. These client responsibilities may be rather minor at first, but they are still of major importance. Not only do they ease the burden for staff, but they are beneficial for the clients as well. They get clients more actively involved in their treatment, care, or education, and this can set the stage for a stronger personal commitment to achieving success. They also give clients a sense of autonomy and personal control, which can offset the negative consequences of feeling weak and helpless.[7]

> This "client responsibility" approach was demonstrated in a Connecticut nursing home. Some of the elderly residents were given more choices and personal responsibility for their life within the institution. They were each given a plant for their room which they had to take care of, they were given a choice of which night they wanted to see a movie, and they were asked for their opinion about how complaints should be handled. A second group of residents (who were of similar age, health, and so on) did not feel responsible for these things because they were told that the staff were responsible: their room plant was watered and cared for by the staff, they were told which night they could see a movie, and they were told that complaints would be handled by the staff. Three weeks later, the "responsibility" residents not only felt more active and happy, but they were evaluated by the staff as more alert, sociable, and involved in activities. Although the "no responsibility" residents had received the same amount of care and attention by the staff, they had become less happy and more debilitated. Two years later, the "responsibility" residents were found to be physically healthier than the other group. Even more dramatic was the fact that twice as many of the "no responsibility" residents had died, compared to the "responsibility" group! Clearly, client responsibility is beneficial to the clients themselves, and is not simply a means for the staff to get out from work.[8]

LIMITING JOB SPILLOVER What people do during their off-duty hours can be critical to coping with on-the-job stress. Because it is so easy for work to spill over into these "nonworking" hours, and even to take over home life, special efforts are needed to protect this private, personal time. As I indicated in the previous chapter, the individual can do a lot to limit this job spillover. However, this individual effort can be greatly strengthened by organizational policies.

Working overtime and being "on call" while off duty are prime examples of job spillover. If these extra hours are optional, then it is up to the individual to decide when enough is enough and to cut back. However, such extra effort is often required by the job, instead of being voluntary, and is actually considered part of the call of duty rather than something above and beyond. In this case, the organization is obligated to specify the limits on these expected "extras." These limitations can refer to the amount of overtime or on-call duty (no more then *x* hours a month, no longer than *x* hours at any one period) or its timing (once a week, weekend duty only once every *x* weeks). Moreover, a policy can be established with respect to staff rotation of these duties, so that the burden is shared equally.

> In one city, the rule was that someone from the psychological emergency team had to accompany police on any calls involving a disturbance or domestic dispute. After one well-publicized incident, in which no member of the team was able to be reached by telephone, a policy was instituted that all team members had to be on call at all hours. As a result, team members began to experience much higher levels of tension and frustration, and a greater disruption of their family life. They never knew what to expect or when, and thus it was impossible ever to know when their off-duty hours were truly off duty. Subsequently, they argued for, and won, a change to a rotation policy in which only two team members were on call at any one time. Not only was this a more efficient and economical policy (since it was rare that more than two people were ever needed), but it put a clear limit on the negative spillover from job to home.

Sometimes rules prohibit staff from socializing with clients or patients outside of the institution. These rules are not intended to make staff act cold and aloof if they happen to see their client at the movies or the grocery store. Rather, the purpose of such a policy is to prevent staff from getting overly involved with their clients, beyond what is necessary in their professional relationship. It is harder for staff to be objective and fair when they are emotionally entangled in a client's life. Furthermore, if the relationship changes from staff-client to one of friends or lovers, then different expectations come into play. For example, we usually allow friends to call us at any time, to ask for special favors, to come visit us at home, and so forth. Should such expectations become part of the staff-client contact, the risk of emotional exhaustion will be greater. After all, how can you ever say no to a friend? Nevertheless, it is important to be able to say no and to set limits on the professional relationship ("We may be partners in solving this problem, but we are not personal friends"). Having an institutional policy to guide and justify these actions can make the whole process an easier one; both staff and recipients know in advance what the limits of the relationship will be.

TAKING TIME OFF The chance to get away from it all can be particularly helpful for someone who is struggling with the stress of burnout. And the organization can provide several different chances. One of these is the "mental health day" (as opposed to sick leave) in which people are given some time off to rest and recharge their batteries. Another is the workshop or training session. Although the main goals of these workshops are to teach and to inspire the staff members, they also serve to get them away from their work for a day or two, sometimes in totally different surroundings.

Perhaps the most common form of time off is the vacation—a period of time when staff people get away from the job by going out of town (or by otherwise being incommunicado). Whatever people do during their vacations, what is most important is that they make a complete break from their job routine so that they can truly relax and unwind. For this reason, one long vacation is often more effective than several short ones. Several weeks are enough time really to get away from the job (both physically and mentally), get a lot of rest, and then get reenergized; a three-day weekend often is not. Organizational flexibility with regard to scheduling these vacations is also very helpful.

The sabbatical is another constructive form of time off, although it is little used outside of educational institutions. A sabbatical refers to an extended period of time (anywhere from a month to a year) when the provider is freed from his or her regular work to do something else that is job enriching. This "something else" can be any number of things, such as traveling to other agencies to study their programs, learning some new skills, doing public relations work for the organization, preparing grant proposals, developing new programs, writing training manuals or other new materials, teaching classes. Such activities get the person out of a rut, provide a welcome change of pace, stimulate new excitement and enthusiasm, and promote professional growth—all the while allowing the person to continue making a useful contribution to the organization.

GETTING HELP · Turning to others for help and support is critical for beating burnout, as I have said throughout this chapter. In addition to informal ways of getting together, several institutional mechanisms can be used as well.

There is strength in numbers, according to the old adage, and that applies to the battle against burnout. Success in instituting changes may only come if people join forces and act as a unified group, rather than as separate individuals. A complaint made by any one person can be easily deflected and turned back against the complainer ("What's the matter with *you*?"). But when there is a group of people with the same complaint, they force attention toward what is going wrong in the work situation and away from individual blame. Whether it be from an organized union, a professional society, or an ad hoc group, this joint effort is often essential for winning the sort of policy changes suggested in this chapter.

Up to this point I have been talking about social support in terms of one's peers or co-workers. However, supervisors are another important source of help and guidance. In my research I have found that burnout rates are lower for staff who have good working relationships with their supervisors and who get support and recognition from them. Supervisors can sensitize staff to the risk of burnout by pointing out problem areas (such as situations where staff are likely to get overextended emotionally) and by alerting them to danger signs (callous jokes or remarks about clients, chronic irritability, increased absenteeism, poor health). If supervisors share their personal experiences, or those of other people they know, they will help prevent new staff from misinterpreting their own reactions as signs of weakness or failure. Supervisors can also provide feedback that is valuable and meaningful to staff, so long as it is clear and specific, and emphasizes the positive instead of just the negative.

When disagreements or conflicts exist between staff and supervisors, it is helpful to set up special group sessions in which gripes can be aired and differences resolved. As opposed to the support groups of peers that I discussed earlier, these sessions would include both staff and supervisors—perhaps separately at first and then together in a joint meeting with a trained leader. One of the benefits of such sessions is that people can get a better sense of how the *other* side sees things, and this insight can help bring about constructive change.

> Diane P. is the social worker described in Chapter 3, who had come to distrust positive feedback from her supervisor because it was always followed by negative criticism. When she (and several others) raised this complaint at an agency retreat, the supervisors were very surprised. Why? Because they had been told that feedback was most effective in the "first positive, then negative" form and had been specifically trained to structure it that way. Once both sides saw what had been happening, they were able to discuss and develop alternative ways of giving feedback, and their feelings of mutual hostility were reduced.

Some organizations offer health insurance coverage for employees' psychological treatment. Other institutions, however, provide specific counseling or therapy services for their employees. These services may be provided in-house (such as the psychological services unit for a police force), or they may be contracted to an outside agency. Counseling is usually provided for a specific problem that is interfering with the employee's work (most commonly, this is alcoholism). However, it is possible to expand the definition of job-related problems to include burnout and to devise counseling or therapy programs for employees who need help in handling it. Supervisors could play an important role in such a program by serving as an early warning system. They can spot early signs of burnout in an employee and may be quicker than he or she is to recognize the problem and try to do something about it.

Although counseling can be helpful, some people are reluctant to try it. There is still a stigma attached to therapy—"Anyone who sees a therapist has got to be crazy." Seeking therapy is believed to be a sign of weakness or failure, and such a belief will inhibit many people from availing themselves of needed help. The use of psychological services will be further reduced if such use can become public knowledge. As an extreme example, the office of the staff psychologist in one police department was put right next door to that of the police chief! The more common concern of employees is that their use of psychological services will be recorded in their personnel file and could not only become known to their supervisors but conceivably be used against them.

If available services are to be utilized, the critical first step is to provide complete confidentiality for the potential users. In organizations that offer mental health insurance benefits, employees' claims should be submitted directly to the insurer and *not* channeled through the organization's personnel office, as is usually done. If treatment is provided in-house, then the office should be located at a distance from the primary work setting and there should be a well-publicized policy that visits to that office will go unrecorded in company files. If confidentiality is not assured, then providers in need of help may not take the step through the therapist's door.

Support services should also be available for the staff person's family, particularly if the job must inevitably disrupt family life (as in the case of police work). It is important that the organization recognize the burden that the job places on the family and try to alleviate it through orientation programs, support groups for spouses and children, social and recreational activities for the families, and family therapy or counseling services (with the same confidentiality given to staff). By giving recognition and help to the family, the organization is, in fact, helping itself. Employees with good, stable family lives are more likely to perform well and are better able to cope with emotional stress. Thus, love and support from others–in this case, one's family–can be a strong line of defense against the deleterious effects of burnout.

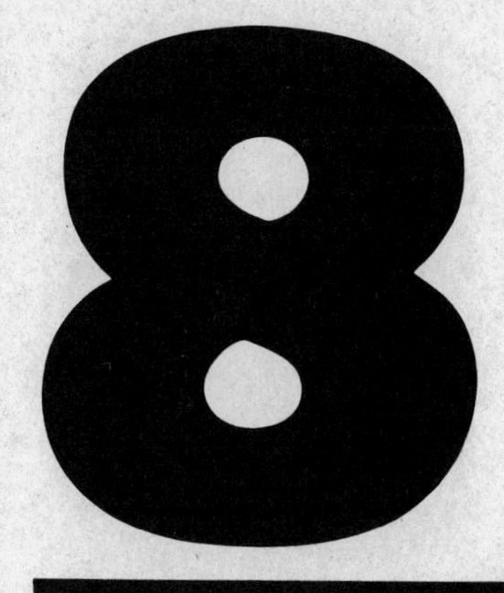

PREVENTING BURNOUT

Early detection: Many psychologists believe themselves to be tough enough to weather emotional travail without support. They may subscribe to a "Lone Ranger" attitude which cuts off avenues for help to the helper. It's a little like avoiding going to a physician with a cut until it has become gangrenous. Get regular check-ups, i.e., scheduled reviews of cases with colleagues or supervisors in which the feelings of the therapist are discussed as well as the technique used.[1]

At Harvard Medical School, Dr. Jerry Avorn developed a new course entitled "Social Theory, Human Values, and the Healing Relationship." This course "weaves practice into theory, its lectures and reading supplemented by class discussions and clinical encounters. . . . Students study how to listen to patients; to understand the special needs of the elderly; to confront dying patients and the impact their death has upon the physician and the family; power conflicts among doctors and the initiation of doctors-to-be into the medical 'guild.' They watch videotapes Dr. Avorn has made of his own patients at Boston's Beth Israel Hospital and conduct similar interviews in class. In papers based on their own clinical experiences, they verbalize not only the patients' feelings but their own. 'It's best

> to reach students when their minds are most open about these issues,' Dr. Avorn says, 'when they haven't been socialized as doctors, and are still willing to admit there's more to medicine than ordering the right lab tests.' "[2]

If an ounce of prevention is worth a pound of cure, then the best way to beat burnout is to keep it from happening in the first place. In other words, take action *before* burnout appears rather than afterward. Instead of suffering through the costs of caring and then trying to recover from them, it makes more sense to try to eliminate them. The costs may be too high ever to be overcome, as we saw in Chapter 5, and thus it is wiser to avoid them altogether.

Prevention is often preached, but it is rarely practiced. People are prone to avoid making any extra efforts until a problem jumps up, knocks them over, and threatens to return worse than before. But dealing with a problem after it has occurred can be quite different than trying to forestall it. For example, trying to change burned-out helpers' cynical view of recipients may be a far more futile effort than trying to maintain the humanized view of recipients that most helpers start with. The inevitable consequence of waiting until there is a problem before doing something, is that what gets done is primarily remedial and rarely preventative.

Not only are few prevention programs ever designed or put into effect, their actual impact is largely unknown. Evaluations of the effectiveness of prevention programs face all the same problems as evaluations of coping strategies. Because of this lack of hard evidence, the proposals for prevention that I will discuss in this chapter are just that—proposals, and not proven principles.

IT'S NEVER TOO EARLY

The key to prevention is early action. The risk of burnout is less likely to become reality if you get a head start on it.

Using Solutions before There Is a Problem

In the last two chapters I talked about a variety of ways to handle burnout. Although these strategies can be used *after* burnout has occurred, as a means of coping with it, they can also be used *before* burnout, as a means of prevention. In other words, do not wait for the problem to arise before using the solutions—use them *now*. Whether they are developing decompression activities or seeking out social support, such strategies make it less likely that there will be a "first time" with burnout. There are several reasons why this should be so. The early use of these techniques will make the job experience less emotionally stressful from the beginning. In addition, early use means that these techniques will become well-practiced parts of your coping style, making you better prepared to handle later problems. When things get tough, it is easier to fall back on something in your regular routine that you already know how to do well, rather than attempt something new and unfamiliar.

Detecting the First Sign

Burnout can be dealt with more effectively in its formative stages than when it is full-blown. Its symptoms are less severe; the problems are minor rather than major; and the individual is still committed, caring, and open to change. Early detection of burnout is thus an important advantage of the preventive approach.

If you are completely burned out, you are sure to know it. However, it is quite possible that someone else will spot the early signs of burnout before you do. Because your focus is directed outward, toward other people and their problems, you pay less attention to what you yourself are doing. You are not likely to notice subtle changes in your mood, your attitudes toward others, or your behavior on the job. And any changes you do notice are likely to be denied or dismissed as being caused by something else.

For these reasons, the best early warning system for burnout lies not in you but in other people. Friends, colleagues, supervisors—all of them may be able to help you recognize what is happening to you and then do something about it. Remember, too, that *you* are the early warning system for someone else. Show concern for your colleagues and be willing to step in with aid and comfort. In helping your peers you also help yourself. First of all, being aware of their behavior can make you more sensitive to your own ("I wonder if *I* do that too?"). Second, your concern helps establish an atmosphere of trust and support, which not only makes the job environment more pleasant, but ensures that you will have people to turn to should your turn come.

The success of such an early warning system depends not only on people's ability to see the warning signs in others, but on their willingness to speak up and say so in a supportive and constructive way. Supervisors are in an excellent position to do this, and so they can be an extremely effective part of any prevention program. The same is true of work colleagues, provided that there is an atmosphere of mutual trust and respect in which feelings and feedback can be shared. There are, however, social forces that work against people's saying something to you about potential problems—they want you to like them, they do not want to be considered nosy busybodies, they may be shy and unassertive (particularly if you appear to be a tough or aloof person who scares people away). For these reasons an early warning system cannot rely on individual initiative alone. Instead, the organization should institute standard reviews, or preburnout "check ups" at periodic intervals (one month after starting the job, then every three months or so). When such reviews are a ritualized and regular procedure for all staff, then no one person has to accept the burden of alerting you to the fact that you are beginning to get singed around the edges.

In addition to individual check ups, regular reviews at the organizational level are an important part of a preventative approach. By discovering what aspects of the job are most clearly linked to the experience of burnout, the organization can institute changes that will improve the job setting and forestall future problems.

> In the course of our research in day-care centers, Ayala Pines and I shared our survey results with all the participating staff.[3] The link we found between burnout and staff-child ratio was not unexpected. However, some of the staff were quite surprised to discover that their emotional exhaustion was related to the unstructured and nondirective quality of their teaching program (a permissive philosophy of which they were very proud). After a series of meetings to discuss the implications of these results, the staff made changes in the structure of the program—changes that were effective, according to a six-month follow-up.[4]

Surveys of organizational staff and recipients are one of the best ways to get needed information about burnout. These surveys would include the Maslach Burnout Inventory as an index of experienced burnout,[5] and questions about job factors that are believed to be implicated in the burnout syndrome. Such questions could be tailored specifically to the particular job setting, or standardized measures could be used. For example, the organizational work environment could be assessed by a Social Climate Scale, as well as by additional questions proposed by the staff.[6] Survey data are used most effectively when staff at *all* organizational levels are involved in contributing questions to be asked, completing the forms, discussing the results, proposing changes, and then carrying them out. This process of shared participation provides staff with a greater sense of autonomy and control—which in itself can reduce burnout. Furthermore, it generates a greater commitment to collaborative problem solving and promotes greater organizational health.[7]

FORWARNED IS FOREARMED

"How come nobody told me it was going to be like this?" This was a constant refrain during my research interviews, and it indicates how ignorant people felt about the emotional stresses of their work. Even if they were knowledgeable and well trained in certain professional skills, they had not been made aware of the potential difficulties of working with people—and thus of the risk of burnout.

> As one attorney who quit after three years of legal services work to go into private practice put it, "I was trained in law, but not in how to work with people who would be my clients. While I could make the transition from theoretical law to practical law, I could not make the transition from idealistic do-gooder to public servant. It was that difficulty in dealing with

people and their personal problems, with having to be a psychiatrist instead of a lawyer, that became the problem for me—not the legal matters per se."[8]

When people do not know ahead of time about the emotional demands of the job, their expectations as they enter that job will be decidedly out of line with reality. The ensuing clash between cherished ideals and the real world is almost certain to lead to burnout. Not only will people feel emotionally exhausted by the demands for which they were unprepared, but they will feel frustrated, disillusioned, and angry (both at others and themselves) because things did not turn out the way they were supposed to be.

According to Dr. Frances J. Storlie of the University of Nevada School of Nursing, the seeds of burnout lie in this conflict between the real and the ideal:

> Burnout requires a susceptible host—that host being the highly idealistic nurse. For many it begins in nursing school. The student is surrounded, nurtured, and protected by teachers, many of whom have had little recent contact with hospitals or direct care of the sick. The ideals the student learns often are unrelated to the real world of health care. When the student is graduated, she reads ads that invite her to work at "the hospital that really cares," or one "that places the patient first," or one where "the patient is our only concern." The young nurse believes that caring matters, that loving and respecting others is what nursing is all about. She hopes to help people to heal, to cure. . . . But often she finds in the hospital setting, "what I was taught" and "what I want to believe" clash with "what really is."[9]

The lack of prior information about sources of emotional stress and the risk of burnout is a striking omission in many training programs. Why should this be? First of all, burnout is considered antithetical to professional ideals. One is not supposed to be emotionally depleted by the work or feel negatively about people. And, as the above quotation suggests, lofty ideals are taught in training programs, not the probable nitty-gritty reality. Second, knowledge about emotional stress is not viewed as being as critical for good performance as other sorts of knowledge or skills. For example, police officers are given lots of training in how to fire a gun but little or no instruction in how to deal with emotional stress. Ironically, most officers will never use their gun while on duty, but they will deal repeatedly with emotionally demanding situations. Similarly, prison guards must work daily with inmates who are difficult to deal with—frustrated, angry, poorly socialized, lacking basic social skills, having poor impulse control, and sometimes physically intimidating. Yet it is rare that the guards' training includes instruction in how to handle the social-psychological problems of their job, although considerable time is spent on security procedures and use of weapons.

A third reason for the absence of prior information has to do with attracting naive recruits into the helping professions. In many cases there is the (erroneous) belief that if people knew how emotionally stressful the career is, they would not choose to enter it. Consequently, little is said about the emotional reality of the work, and sometimes there is a deliberate misrepresentation of the job.

> For example, some people in legal services have acknowledged that they do not tell the whole truth to prospective employees: "We aren't always completely honest with people—we know that. But if they really knew what this job is like, they wouldn't bother to sign up. It's better to hook them first, get them into the job, and then let them find out later." A similar "get them first, tell them later" argument has been made by correctional staff.

In contrast, my own position is that the more prior information there is about burnout, the better. People should have more accurate expectations about the work they are getting into before they actually start on the job. If they did, there would be fewer unpleasant "surprises" or "reality shocks" that shatter their ideals or lead them to consider themselves as total failures. Some people might realize that this is the wrong career for them and drop out *before* entering it, rather than afterward. Thus, the costs associated with attrition and turnover may be greatly reduced by providing realistic previews of the job—a conclusion that is supported by research studies.[10] Furthermore, prior knowledge about burnout will make people better able to recognize it in its early stages, either in themselves or in others. Greater awareness of the risk of burnout can also lead people to be better prepared for it ahead of time. They can anticipate sources of emotional stress before they occur and develop plans for how to handle them. They will have a clearer sense of the personal skills and the social support they will need to do their job successfully and can take steps to get them before any problems arise.

Information about burnout—its causes and consequences, and appropriate coping strategies—should be a required part of the training curriculum for any people-work profession. Such information will be especially influential if the faculty of the training program actually practice the professional behaviors and balanced life-style that they preach. For example, medical school faculty who warn against sacrificing family life to career should not be modeling a seventy-hour workweek themselves. In addition to information presented in courses, social support groups could also be started during the training program. Teaching people early in their career to share ideas and feelings with others, to give and receive feedback, and to help each other out, will enable them to have more effective relations with their actual work colleagues. Even though burnout is not an inevitable experience for everyone, it *is* a potential risk, and knowledge of that risk (and a healthy respect for it) will lessen the possibility that a potential risk will become a probable fate.

THE PREPARED MIND (AND HEART)

"Be prepared" is a motto that applies as much to burnout as to Boy Scouts. And the preparation that is most needed is training in interpersonal skills. While professional providers are often well trained in certain healing, teaching, or service skills, they are often not well equipped to handle repeated, intense, emotional contacts with people. This point is illustrated by the attorney quoted earlier who felt prepared to deal with legal problems but not people problems. Although most helpers want training in interpersonal skills, few ever get it.

The Need to Learn Interpersonal Skills

Surprisingly, interpersonal skills are often not recognized as a major necessity for providers. They are considered secondary to other professional skills–extras rather than essentials, the "icing on the cake" rather than the cake itself. "It's nice if you have it, but you don't really need it" is often the prevailing wisdom.

> The attitude of several physicians that I interviewed is that the competent practice of medicine is all they need to know to be successful in their career. As far as they are concerned, training in interpersonal skills simply means knowing how to make "small talk" with their patients. Such a skill is viewed as pleasant, but it is not considered central to medical care. As one physician put it, "If that's what patients want, they should go see a priest."

In my opinion, this viewpoint is sadly in error, for it trivializes an essential aspect of the relationship between provider and recipient. It fails to recognize that both of them are human beings whose personal attitudes and feelings can affect not only the delivery of care, but also how and even whether it is accepted.

Even when interpersonal skills are considered important, it is often assumed that they cannot be taught. In part, this is because of the belief that these skills reflect basic personality, and either people have them or they don't. In other words, such skills are considered a natural "gift" or talent that some people just happen to be blessed with. According to this view, teachers (doctors, therapists, and others) are born, not made.

A very different argument against skills training is the notion that interpersonal skills can only be acquired through on-the-job experience–not in formal classes. According to this view, interpersonal "savvy" can only be learned in the school of hard knocks. Direct experience is indeed a better teacher than textbook descriptions, but leaving these experiences up to chance does not guarantee that their effects will always be positive. Some people will learn from their experiences, but others will not; and of those who do learn, some will learn quickly but others will not learn until much later. Leaving this learning process up to chance also means that people will be picking up interpersonal skills by trial and error, and since the errors are often at the client's expense, this strategy is a costly one. Moreover, the skills providers do happen to pick up may not be the optimal ones. Specific skills and tactics are best utilized when developed as part of more general strategies and guided by explicit goals and objectives, and not when developed on the pragmatic basis of "if it works, keep doing it."

Experiential learning is not limited to the actual job, however, but can be a key part of professional training programs. Within this context, the virtues of direct experience can be combined with more structured situations in which there is both guidance and feedback. A critical necessity for such training is books or training manuals that deal with the *technique* of helping (and not just with philosophy and abstract analysis). Such books are relatively few and have only begun to appear in the last few years; clearly, many more are needed.[11] The techniques that are taught must then actually be tried out by the trainees. Role playing and practice sessions are especially effective in getting trainees to rehearse these techniques and become skilled in their use. An example of this approach is a training program entitled *Helping Skills*, which is designed to teach some basic helping techniques to a wide range of people workers.[12]

At later stages of training a supervised internship (in which the trainee's work with people is observed and recorded for later evaluation and feedback) can help develop interpersonal skills even further.

> At Children's Hospital of Los Angeles, pediatric interns were videotaped while they were seeing patients in one of the clinics. Analyses of these videotapes revealed specific strengths and weaknesses in the interns' behavior toward both the child and the parent. "Interns seldom introduced the visit with social talk, sometimes failed to greet the family or say farewell, and did not always make the mother physically comfortable. Interns generally were patient and concerned, but often they were insensitive to aspects of the situation such as emotions expressed by the mother, or the presence of other family members during the visit. Although rarely critical, interns were also rarely empathetic or supportive. Communication skills were sometimes poor. Jargon and leading questions were sometimes used, and the mother did not always have ample opportunity for her questions to be answered. However, information was usually given clearly. Interns paid little attention to psychosocial issues, rarely discussing topics such as behavior and the home environment."[13] Given this information, the medical faculty could pinpoint those areas in which additional interpersonal skills were needed and revise the training program accordingly. Many medical schools and residency programs now use videotape feedback to teach interviewing skills to physicians. Although the best way to use such video-

tapes has not been established, they clearly have the potential to be highly effective teaching devices.

RECIPIENTS AS TEACHERS Another teaching device that is rarely, if ever, used is to have actual clients or patients involved in training providers.[14] While providers may "practice" their newly acquired skills on recipients during an internship, they do not regard them as potential resources. Yet the knowledge and insight that come from understanding the recipient's view of the helping process could be invaluable. The expectations recipients have, the sources of confusion or conflict, the things they like or dislike about a particular practitioner's interpersonal style—such information could provide guidance for training programs by indicating where the training is on target and by pointing out problem areas that have not been addressed. Recipients could "teach" in a variety of ways—participating in class discussions, role playing, commenting on case conferences or practice sessions, and so forth. In addition to current recipients, *former* recipients might also play an important role in training programs. Not only do they know what things were like when they needed help, but they can evaluate these experiences in comparison to their current life situation. Moreover, they may be better able to articulate what recipients are actually thinking and feeling about the helping relationship. Current and former recipients are beginning to play a more active and responsible role in various treatment programs, such as the innovative self-help project for mental patients at the Elgin Mental Health center in Illinois.[15] Perhaps training programs could take a cue from such projects and develop new roles for recipients in the teaching process.

What Interpersonal Skills Need to Be Learned

The chronic, day-in-and-day-out emotional stresses of the job are most strongly linked to burnout—not the occasional crises or emergencies. Ironically, while people workers are often taught crisis skills, they are rarely trained in the common, "garden variety" skills that they need to use routinely. The importance of such everyday skills may be underestimated because they seem like basic abilities that are shared by all human beings ("Everybody knows how to talk to people, to get along with them, right? They do it all the time at home and with their friends, so they should just do the same things at work"). However, people's personal experiences rarely prepare them for continuous, emotionally intense encounters with clients, which are the reality of the job, and so special skills training is indeed necessary.

The interpersonal skills that I will mention here do not constitute a complete and comprehensive list, but are examples of the sorts of things that many providers wish they knew how to do well. I will not attempt to present a general procedure for learning these skills, however, since I believe that an effective training program has to be tailored to the specific needs and demands of the particular profession. Rather, my aim is simply to call attention to the importance of these skills and to suggest that programs be developed to teach them within the context of professional education.

HOW TO START, STOP, AND KEEP THINGS GOING Just like true love, the course of helping relationships does not always run smooth. Getting things started on the right foot often depends on how you greet the other person, whether there is any initial social talk to reduce tension and "break the ice," how often you use his or her name, whether you give off cues of impatience ("Make it quick—there are other people waiting to see me"), and so forth. Similarly, bringing things to a successful halt depends on whether you interrupt the person (and how you do so), how you announce that time is up, whether you evaluate the progress that has been made, how you say good-bye and so on. Just as important as the words you use are the messages you convey through your body language (looking directly at the other person, nodding your head, smiling). Videotapes of interactions between clients and practitioners who are successful and well liked would provide ideas on what words and gestures are most effective in establishing good rapport. Commentary about the videotapes by both the clients and the practitioner involved would also be especially helpful.

In many cases, contact with clients covers more than one session and centers on the completion of certain goals. For example, a physician tries to get a patient to follow a prescribed treatment or return for regular follow-up visits. Or a parole officer tries to get a former prisoner to make (and keep) an appointment with an employment agency. Or a social worker tries to get a parent to make regular child support payments or take his or her child to a dentist for needed treatment. Or a teacher tries to get a student to turn in assigned homework. Or a practitioner tries to get patients to pay their bills. If you are in such a situation, you are automatically stuck with having to "nag" people—a task that is uncomfortable at best and often frustrating and infuriating. There are no easy solutions for this age-old problem, but you can learn new ways to be persuasive with people.

> A continuing problem for physicians has been "patient noncompliance"—that is, patients' failure to follow medical advice or prescribed treatment. One solution is to teach physicians how to communicate clearly with patients, without using jargon and complicated terminology. Another strategy is to get someone else on the health care team to be responsible for explaining procedures to patients. A different approach is to take the process of one-sided communications from physician (superior) to patient (inferior) and change it to one of negotiation between two active and equal participants. "Conflict exists between the physician, who wishes to have his patient follow directions exactly as he prescribes, and the patient, who wishes to get away with as little as possible and still maintain his health. Clinical negotiation is a deliberate attempt to reduce this conflict

by pinpointing areas of agreement and disagreement. Each party gets an understanding of the other's viewpoint and can respond."[16] Strategies of patient-physician negotiation, such as the ones used at Temple University Hospital in Philadelphia, have been found effective.

HOW TO DEAL WITH DIFFERENT PEOPLE The infinite variety of human beings is what makes working with people so interesting, exciting, and challenging. It is also what makes it so difficult at times. The approach that a practitioner uses with one client (patient, student, or whoever) may not work with someone else because of differences in sex, age, cultural background, personality, values, attitudes, and so forth. For example, if the hospital patient is an elderly Italian immigrant, he may expect the doctor to make all of the decisions for him and thus will be uncomfortable with the active participation role thrust upon him by the negotiation process. Or a student who is very shy may not respond to the teacher's offer to help with the assignment, even though such help is desired. Dealing with people who are rude, belligerent, and even threatening requires different skills than working with people who rarely talk and do not look you in the eye.

Although practitioners often long for a single strategy that will work well with everybody ("Just tell me the best way to do it, and I'll do it"), the truth is that they need to have several different strategies in their hip pocket, ready to be used when appropriate. They can learn many of these from their more experienced colleagues, who can alert them to the sorts of people they are likely to see and share some professional tips on what to say and do with them. "The best thing to do with this kind of guy is to set up very concrete goals at the beginning of the session–like, 'we're going to sit here for an hour, and we're going to discuss what's happening with your kids.'" Information and comments from recipients could also be especially valuable here, since they could point out to practitioners what interpersonal style they respond to best.

HOW TO TALK ABOUT UNPOPULAR TOPICS All too often in helping relationships what needs to be said is what one person does not want to say and the other does not want to hear. Practitioners dread these difficult moments, and it is here, more than anywhere else, that they express a need for additional interpersonal skills. Without them, they either do the job badly or avoid it completely, hoping that somehow, someone else will do the dirty work.

The topics that are the most difficult to handle are: how to ask tough questions, how to discuss sensitive issues, and how to deliver bad news. Tough questions include those that are embarrassing (for the client or the staff person), that are likely to reveal a client's failure or inadequacies, that may uncover incriminating information, or that could provoke anger or emotional distress. Sensitive issues include the reasons for a person's failure; the blame for a criminal act; and almost anything having to do with sex, money, or death. However, being the bearer of bad tidings is the one thing that people workers dread most. Having to say no, denying a request, terminating a contract, or saying that no more services or treatments are available, are all instances in which the provider stops providing. Telling people that they failed, or that they will be punished, or that their problems are getting worse, or that they are dying–in these cases, the bad news focuses on the recipient's experience. No matter what the unpopular topic happens to be, it is enormously stressful and emotionally taxing to have to deal with it. Special skills training for this problem would go a long way toward alleviating the emotional exhaustion of burnout.

A FINAL ANALYSIS

I have said many different things in this book about what burnout is and what to do about it—so many things, in fact, that it may appear to be a complex jumble of causes and effects, problems and solutions, rather than a neat and simple package. However, there is order in this complexity, not chaos. Several key themes run throughout the book and tie together its various parts.

LEVELS OF ANALYSIS

In my discussion of burnout I have first considered contributing factors (Chapters 2-4), then resultant effects (Chapter 5), and finally potential solutions (Chapters 6-8). However, a crosscutting theme is the level at which each of these phenomena takes place: individual, interpersonal, and institutional. What is important to recognize here is that burnout occurs at *all* of these levels, and not just one. It is not simply a matter of certain types of individuals who cannot handle the job, nor is it simply the nature of the job irrespective of the people who perform it. Rather, I would argue that there is a complex interaction between individual, interpersonal, and institutional factors, and that all of them have to be taken into account. The pattern of this interaction is still unclear—we do not yet know the relative importance of each dimension to answer questions such as, "Does the nature of the job have a greater impact than the individual's personality, or vice versa?" Nor do we know just how one dimension influences the other. Nevertheless, an awareness of these three levels at which burnout occurs can help inform our understanding of it.

Individual

The question that is being addressed at this level is, "What role does the *person* play in burnout?" In other words, what are the personal causes of burnout, the personal effects, and the personal solutions to it? As we saw in Chapter 4, individual contributions to burnout include certain personality traits and background characteristics. Burnout will be more likely if the person is younger, less mature, and less self-confident; is impulsive and impatient; has no family commitments but needs other people who can provide approval and affection; has goals and expectations that are not in tune with reality. At the individual level, burnout results in both physical and psychological dysfunction. Exhaustion and illness, depression and irritability, increased use of alcohol and drugs—these are some of the personal costs. However, the individual can do a wide range of things to combat burnout, as we saw in Chapter 6. These personal strategies involve various ways of changing one's style of work and of taking better care of oneself.

Interpersonal

At this level the question is, "What role do *other people* play in burnout?" That is, what is the impact of the social situation surrounding the individual? The nature of one's involvement with recipients can precipitate burnout, as discussed in Chapter 2. The feelings and tensions that are part of the helping relationship, the negative focus on problems, the emotional strain of empathy—all of these factors make the individual vulnerable to burnout. Another contributing factor at the interpersonal level is difficulties with co-workers and with supervisors (see Chapter 3). The interpersonal effects of burnout are seen most clearly in the relations with recipients: a decrease in time spent with them, an increase in callous and insensitive behavior, and a deterioration in the overall quality of care. These negative effects can hurt one's family and friends as well. In Chapter 7 I discussed interpersonal coping techniques, in all of which the individual draws on the resources of other people and joins forces with them in the battle against burnout.

Institutional

The question being raised here is, "What role does the *organization* play in burnout?" In other words, what happens at the level of the job setting, over and above the individuals who staff it? There are many ways in which the institution contributes to burnout, including excessive case loads, restrictive regulations, and poor management (see Chapter 3). The effects of burnout at the institutional level are reflected in high rates of absenteeism, turnover, and complaints about staff performance. There are, however, many institutional strategies for handling burnout, as mentioned in Chapters 7 and 8: redesigning jobs, changing organizational policies, devising explicit structures and contracts, establishing flexible leaves and support services, and improving the training programs for staff.

POWER VERSUS POWERLESSNESS

Another key theme that appears throughout this book is the importance of autonomy and personal control. Burnout is a greater risk whenever people feel powerless—when they feel trapped by other people's demands, when they are weak and unassertive in their personal style, when they feel held down and boxed in by institutional regulations and endless demands of those they serve. They have the sense that they are at the mercy of the situation and that there is nothing they can do about it. "It's hopeless; you can't change things; it's bigger than all of us, so why bother trying?" If our behavior does not control relevant contingent outcomes, we learn to believe that we are helpless and our situation is hopeless.

Many of the strategies for coping with burnout are, in fact, strategies for personal power. They are ways in which the individual exerts some active control in a situation, rather than just passively acquiescing to it. The person changes the work routine, redefines goals, utilizes downshifts, takes breaks, seeks out positive feedback, engages in decompression activities, and so forth. All of these actions involve *choice* and *initiative*—the hallmarks of freedom and autonomy. The individual considers alternative possibilities, decides which ones to carry out, and then *acts.* The personal consequences of such personal control are very positive, in terms of enhanced confidence and self-esteem, and a greater sense of power and independence. Even when the actions are fairly minor ones, these benefits still accrue (as we saw with patients in the nursing home example in Chapter 7). Although it is rare that someone has direct control over everything in the work situation, the individual practitioner probably has more personal power than he or she acknowledges. By wiggling around in the job and finding out what can change and what cannot, the practitioner can counteract the helplessness and "the-hell-with-it-all" attitude associated with burnout.

Often when workers are dissatisfied with the quality of life on their jobs, they strike for more pay. In part, they may be doing so as a protest against feeling powerless or unappreciated, or because they feel that now they are simply in it for the money. Organizations must recognize the important role that work plays in giving a worker a sense of identity and self-worth. The institution must strive actively to do all in its power to enhance each worker's sense of personal accomplishment and the feeling that "I work at this job because it is what I *want* to do, and not because I have to."

BALANCE VERSUS BURNOUT

If all the knowledge and advice about how to beat burnout could be summed up in one word, that word would be *balance.* Balance between giving and getting, balance between stress and calm, balance between work and home–these stand in clear contrast to the overload, understaffing, overcommitment, and other imbalances of burnout. "To give and give and give until there is nothing left to give anymore" means that one has failed to replenish one's resources. Unless more fuel is brought to the fire it will eventually use up all that was there to start the flame–and then die out. In a similar way, unless one has fueled oneself (with knowledge, rewards, strength), the fires of compassion can be all-consuming, leaving nothing but emotional ashes.

The basic message here is that giving *of* yourself must be balanced with giving *to* yourself. Making yourself strong, knowledgeable, and in good spirits makes you a better provider for those in need. Thus, it is sensible (not selfish) to take time off to relax, to seek out advice and support from others, to mix periods of undemanding work among the more stressful ones, to stop job spillover into your home life, and so forth. If you recognize your limits and acknowledge your needs, you will be less likely to overextend yourself to the point of no recovery. This does not mean that you cannot go overboard at times, when you think it is necessary; however, if you do so, then you need to do something extra to recuperate and restore yourself.

Detached Concern

This theme of balance is also at the heart of "detached concern"–that ideal blend of compassion and objectivity that many people workers strive for. The provider is genuinely concerned about people's well-being but has some psychological distance from their problems. There is neither too much involvement nor too little. The provider deals with emotionally arousing situations without getting overwhelmed by them.

In detached concern there is the recognition that, in different ways, both distance and closeness can help people deal with the emotional demands of the helping relationship. By being close and concerned the provider sees the recipient as a fellow human being (instead of an anonymous statistic), has a more sensitive understanding of the problems that person is facing, and is personally motivated to help. On the other hand, by being distant and detached the caregiver appraises the problems objectively (instead of being blinded by personal biases and feelings), implements solutions in an orderly and rational way, and is straightforward in assessing their success (or failure). Thus, detachment and concern complement each other, with the benefits of one offsetting the potential pitfalls of the other. To provide the best—whether it be service, care, treatment, or education—the helper should use *both* objective detachment and sensitive concern, rather than choosing one over the other.

Although this balanced state of detached concern may sound good in theory, it is not always clear how to achieve it in practice. The skills that are necessary to maintain professional detachment may be quite different from those used to maintain interested concern—in fact, they may even be in conflict. Indeed, some practitioners talk about moving back and forth between these two states, rather than trying to combine them.

Nevertheless, in spite of the inherent difficulties in achieving detached concern, it is still a goal worth striving for. Many of the skills and coping techniques discussed in this book can be considered as means toward that end. In time, we may know better which techniques are the most effective ones; someday soon, there may even be formal programs to provide regular training in detached concern for professional providers of help to the many people who need their help.

To the age-old question, "Who will help the helper?" my answer is that I hope this book has. By providing needed knowledge and by pointing out paths to needed change it represents a step in the direction of a better future—a future in which burnout poses less of a threat to people workers than it does now. I am enough of an optimist to believe that burnout *can* be beaten, and that it is not an inevitable price that people must pay for caring. To the extent that we overcome, reduce, or prevent burnout in any person subject to its destructive force, we help bind that person to a network of more meaningful social and professional relationships—a network that reaffirms and bolsters the very foundation of the human connection.

APPENDIX: TECHNIQUES FOR STRESS MANAGEMENT

STRESS MANAGEMENT SKILLS

Two basic skills are of central importance in a stress management program. They are deep muscle relaxation and mental relaxation. The technique that follows is one we at the Stanford Heart Disease Prevention Program have devised and find most useful in our work. Though it is by no means the only effective relaxation method, it is easily learned and practiced. (Two points of caution are important: Under *no* circumstances should anyone on blood-pressure-lowering medications stop using these medications after starting relaxation methods. You may find that your pill dosage may be reduced but this should be done in close cooperation with your physician. Furthermore, if you have a history of prior serious mental illness, do *not* begin a program of stress management without consulting with your doctor.)

Deep Muscle Relaxation Drill

1. Find as quiet an environment as possible. Lie on your back in a comfortable position or sit comfortably. Close your eyes.

2. For right-handed people, begin by physically tensing the right hand for an instant, then relax and let it go loose. Tell it to be heavy and warm. Continue with the rest of the right side of the body, moving up to forearm, upper arm, shoulder, then down to the foot, lower leg, and upper leg. Next, follow the same procedure on the left side of the body. (If you are left-handed, begin the procedure with the left hand and continue.) The hands, arms, and legs are now relaxed, heavy, and warm. Wait for these feelings. (After mastering the technique, you will not need to tense the muscles before relaxing them.)

3. Next, relax the muscles of the hips and let a wave of relaxation pass up from the abdomen to the chest. Do not tense these muscles. Tell them to be heavy and warm. Your breathing will come more from the diaphragm and will be slower. Wait for this breathing change.

4. Now let the wave of relaxation continue into the shoulders, neck, jaw, and the muscles of the face. Pay special attention to the muscles controlling the eyes and forehead. Finish the drill by telling your forehead to feel cool.

Practice this drill twice daily; fifteen to twenty minutes is ideal (but even three minutes is better than nothing when circumstances do not permit a longer session). Practice before meals or no sooner than one hour after meals. You can also practice before an anticipated stress experience but no more frequently than four times a day.

With practice you will learn to attain deep muscle relaxation—the feeling of heavy, warm, inert muscles and a cool forehead—in as short a time as two minutes. An Instant Relaxation Drill, to be described later, is designed for use before and during stressful periods in the course of your normal activities when longer relaxation periods are clearly not practical.

If you are not sure whether or not you are relaxed, ask another person to raise your arm or leg about six inches and then let go. If it drops as a dead weight, your muscles are relaxed. Jerky resistance indicates that muscle tension is still present. The benefits of deep muscle relaxation are many: lowered pulse rate and blood pressure, lowered breathing rate, decreased bodily oxygen consumption, and a general feeling of calmness and tranquility.

MENTAL RELAXATION

When you have learned to achieve at least a partial state of deep muscle relaxation, you are ready for the next step in relaxation—clearing your mind of stressful thoughts and worries through mastery of the Mental Relaxation Drill that follows.

Mental Relaxation Drill

After entering a state of deep muscle relaxation, you are ready to begin the mind-clearing process that deepens the relaxation state. Your eyes are closed and your forehead is cool.

1. Enter a passive state; let thoughts flow through your head.

2. If thoughts recur, respond by saying "no" under your breath.

3. Imagine a calm blue sky or sea or any blue area or object without detail (with your eyes closed). Try to see the color blue (which has been found to be a particularly relaxing color).

4. Become aware of your slow, natural breathing. Follow each breath as you inhale and exhale.

5. If you still do not feel calm and restful, you may find it helpful to use a repeated, soothing word (such as love or God) or less symbolic word (such as *now* or *breath*). If you find that using a word distracts you, try using a sound (such as "ah"). Think of the word or sound silently, preferably during exhalation. Always remind yourself to keep the muscles of the face, eyes, and forehead loose, and to keep your forehead cool.

The Deep Muscle Relaxation and Mental Relaxation drills are interactive and should ordinarily be done together. Once you have learned both drills, simply combine them. Practice this combined Deep Muscle/Mental Relaxation Drill twice daily.

In our stress management classes at the Stanford Heart Disease Prevention Program, we have found that using the Deep Muscle/Mental Relaxation Drill twice daily, combined with occasional use of an instant relaxation method (to be described later), is sufficient to produce a gratifying lowering of blood pressure in most patients. Among that group, those who practiced the relaxation techniques most regularly received the greatest benefits. Other research workers, in this country and in England, have also reported beneficial results in treating high blood pressure through the use of relaxation methods.

In the beginning, until these skills are mastered, frequent practice is the best plan. It may take a few weeks to reach the goal of not only decreased respiration and lowered blood pressure but also the general feeling of tranquility that you gain from better stress management.

IMAGERY TRAINING

Imagery training is a useful method to assist you in the Deep Muscle Relaxation and Mental Relaxation drills. Imagery training breaks down mental blocks to the use of your imagination. For people who are out of touch with their bodies, deep muscle relaxation is sometimes difficult to learn. Test yourself. Think of your left ear; make it feel warm. Imagine your right calf muscle as feeling warm and heavy. Now try two harder tests. Imagine the left leg is heavier than the right leg. Reverse the feelings. If you can do these tests easily, you should find it relatively easy to achieve deep muscle relaxation. If you cannot, you will benefit from the following muscle-finding drills.

Drills for Muscle Finding

1. Lie comfortably on your back in a quiet room. Become passive.

2. Tense all the muscles of your body for about five seconds, then let them go as limp as you can. Notice the difference in feeling.

3. Repeat this, but now exhale your breath slowly during the total body relaxation. This will help create a limp, relaxed state.

4. Try tensing and "letting go" of individual sets of muscles: hand, arm, foot, lower leg, upper leg, buttocks, neck, jaws, mouth, face, and forehead.

If you are uncertain whether or not you are relaxed, ask a helper to judge your muscle tension by picking up your arm about six inches and letting it drop. After a few weeks' practice, almost everyone will have been able to reduce muscle tension to zero (on a scale of 4 to 0).

Relaxation tapes for home playing may be helpful for those who have difficulty with unaided self-instruction, or you can tape your own instructions for these drills.

IMAGERY TRAINING FOR MENTAL RELAXATION

Even though you do well in deep muscle relaxation, intrusive, racing thoughts can prevent you from reaching a stage of complete muscle relaxation as well as complete mental relaxation. Still, you may find this stage of partial deep muscle relaxation and free association of ideas rather pleasant. It can be a time for surprisingly effective problem solving. To achieve complete mental relaxation, it is helpful to incorporate imagery training into your relaxation drills by following these steps.

Imagery Drill for Mental Relaxation

1. Bring yourself as deeply into the Deep Muscle/Mental Relaxation Drill as possible. Assuming that intrusive or racing thoughts remain a problem, read on.

2. Use the following two methods of "thought stopping":

a. When a thought returns too frequently or persists, say "no" out loud. If it returns, say "no" again. Use this self-command repeatedly over a five- to ten-minute period, while remaining in the deep muscle relaxation and mental relaxation states.

b. If the verbal commands to stop seem to decrease the frequency of the recurrent intrusions, then change to a silent "no" when an unwanted, recurrent, or persistent thought prevents your entry into complete mind clearing. When a further reduction in active thinking occurs, you are ready to continue.

3. Imagine a pleasant scene, such as a mountain lake, a calm ocean, a blue sky with drifting white clouds. Focus on this scene to replace the previous intrusive, racing thoughts.

4. When this succeeds, let the pleasant scene fade and enter the final stages of the drill.

5. Let a gray or black "nothingness" be the image before your closed eyes. Ignore any visual detail.

6. Finally, let blue colors drift in, often as patches. When they come, hold on to the particular feeling that lets the blue colors in. When you are at this point, you have usually reached zero muscle tension and complete mental relaxation.

INSTANT RELAXATION

After you have achieved a satisfactory degree of success in deep muscle relaxation and mental relaxation, you should be able to enter partially into deep muscle relaxation and mental relaxation states within thirty seconds to three minutes. You are now ready to practice instant relaxation.

Instant Relaxation Drill

1. Sit comfortably. (You can also learn to do this while standing, waiting in line, or just prior to an anticipated stressful event.)

2. Draw in a deep breath and hold it for five seconds (count to five slowly), exhale slowly and tell all your muscles to relax. Repeat this two or three times to become more completely relaxed.

3. If circumstances permit, imagine a pleasant thought ("I am learning how to relax") or a pleasant scene (a calm ocean, a mountain stream, etc.).

Develop cuing systems to remind yourself to use this drill (for example, any time you become impatient over having to wait). The Instant Relaxation Drill takes from thirty to sixty seconds. In most stress circumstances, you can benefit from using either a Deep Muscle/Mental Relaxation Drill or an Instant Relaxation Drill. Each can be used when you are consciously attacking a specific, recurrent stress that you have identified. Each can also be used as a refresher interspersed in your daily routine.

CHAPTER NOTES

Unless otherwise noted, all individual quotations are drawn from research interviews that I conducted or from personal letters that were sent to me. To protect people's privacy, all names and identifying information have been changed.

PROLOGUE

[1] Printed with the permission of Ron Petrillo.

CHAPTER 1–THE BURNOUT SYNDROME

[1] Lief, H. I., & Fox, R. C. Training for "detached concern" in medical students, In H. I. Lief, V. F. Lief, & N. R. Lief (Eds.), *The psychological basis of medical practice.* New York: Harper & Row, 1963.

[2] Maslach, C. *"Detached concern" in health and social service professions.* Paper presented at the annual convention of the American Psychological Association, Montreal, August 1973.

[3] Maslach, C. Burned-out. *Human Behavior,* 1976, *5*(9), 16-22.

[4] Maslach, C., & Pines, A. The burn-out syndrome in the day care setting. *Child Care Quarterly,* 1977, *6,* 100-113.

Pines, A., & Maslach, C. Combatting staff burnout in a day care center: A case study. *Child Care Quarterly,* 1980, *9,* 5-16.

[5] Pines, A., & Maslach, C. Characteristics of staff burn-out in mental health settings. *Hospital and Community Psychiatry,* 1978, *29,* 233-237.

[6] Maslach, C., & Jackson, S. E. Lawyer burn-out. *Barrister,* 1978, *5*(2), 8; 52-54.

[7] Maslach, C., & Jackson, S. E. Burned-out cops and their families. *Psychology Today,* 1979, *12*(12), 59-62.

Jackson, S. E., & Maslach, C. After-effects of job-related stress: Families as victims. *Journal of Occupational Behaviour,* 1982, *3.*

[8] Maslach, C., & Jackson, S. E. Burnout in health professions: A social psychological analysis. In G. Sanders & J. Suls (Eds.), *Social psychology of health and illness.* Hillsdale, N.J.: Lawrence Erlbaum, 1982, in press.

Jackson, S. E., & Maslach, C. *Burnout and the medical work environment.* Unpublished manuscript, 1982.

[9] Maslach, C., Jackson, S. E., & Barad, C. B. *Patterns of burnout among a national sample of public contact workers.* Unpublished manuscript, 1982.

[10] Readers who are interested in reviewing the psychometric properties of the MBI and the factor analysis that is the basis for the three subscales, are referred to: Maslach, C., & Jackson, S. E. The measurement of experienced burnout. *Journal of Occupational Behaviour,* 1981, *2,* 99-113; Maslach, C., & Jackson, S. E. *The Maslach Burnout Inventory* ("Human Services Survey"). (Research Ed.). Palo Alto, Calif.: Consulting Psychologists Press, 1981.

[11] Adapted from Maslach, C., & Jackson, S. E. *The Maslach Burnout Inventory* ("Human Services Survey"). Research Edition. Palo Alto, Calif.: Consulting Psychologists Press, 1981. Copyright © 1981 by Consulting Psychologists Press, Inc. All rights reserved. For information about obtaining test forms and a user's manual, please write to the publisher at 577 College Avenue, Palo Alto, California 94306.

[12] Maslach, C. Burnout: A social psychological analysis. In J. W. Jones (Ed.), *The burnout syndrome: Current research, theory, interventions.* Park Ridge, Ill.: London House Press, 1981.

Maslach, C. Job burn-out: How people cope. *Public Welfare,* 1978, *36*(2), 56-58.

Maslach, C. The client role in staff burn-out. *Journal of Social Issues,* 1978, *34*(4), 111-124.

Maslach, C., & Pines, A. Burnout: The loss of human caring. In A. Pines & C. Maslach (Eds.), *Experiencing social psychology.* New York: Knopf, 1979.

Maslach, C. The burn-out syndrome and patient care. In C. A. Garfield (Ed.), *Stress and survival: The emotional realities of life-threatening illness.* St. Louis: Mosby, 1979.

Maslach, C. Understanding burnout: Definitional issues in analyzing a complex phenomenon. In W. S. Paine (Ed.), *Job Stress and Burnout.* Beverly Hills, Calif.: Sage Publications, 1982.

[13]Ross, L. The intuitive psychologist and his shortcomings: Distortions in the attribution process. In L. Berkowitz (Ed.), *Advances in experimental social psychology.* (Vol. 10). New York: Academic Press, 1977.

[14]Ryan, W. *Blaming the victim.* New York: Pantheon, 1971.

CHAPTER 2–INVOLVEMENT WITH PEOPLE AS A SOURCE OF BURNOUT

[1]Letter appearing in the Dear Abby column of the *San Francisco Chronicle,* November 12, 1976. Copyright, 1976, Universal Press Syndicate. Reprinted with permission. All rights reserved.

[2]Roth, J. A. Some contingencies of the moral evaluation and control of clientele: The case of the hospital emergency service. *American Journal of Sociology,* 1972, *77,* 839-856.

[3]Wills, T. A. Perceptions of clients by professional helpers. *Psychological Bulletin,* 1978, *85,* 968-1000.

[4]Copyright 1975, National Association of Social Workers, Inc. Reprinted with permission from Stromer, W. F. *Social Work,* 1975, *20*(3), 238-239.

[5]Jupiter, H. Scary times at the S.F. Welfare Office. *San Francisco Chronicle,* January 17, 1975. © San Francisco Chronicle, 1975. Reprinted by permission.

[6]Koocher, G. P. Adjustment and coping strategies among the caretakers of cancer patients. Reprinted from *Social Work in Health Care,* 1979, *5*(2), 145-150. © 1979 by The Haworth Press, Inc. Used by permission. All rights reserved.

[7]Saul, E. V., & Kass, T. S. Study of anticipated anxiety in a medical school setting. *Journal of Medical Education,* 1969, *44,* 526-532.

[8]Maltsberger, T., & Buie, D. H. Countertransference hate in the treatment of suicidal patients. *Archives of General Psychiatry,* 1974, *30,* 625-633.

[9]Koocher, G. P. Pediatric cancer: Psychosocial problems and the high costs of helping. *Journal of Clinical Child Psychology,* 1980, *10,* 2-5. Used by permission of the publisher.

[10]Westerhouse, M. A. *The effects of tenure, role conflict, and role conflict resolution on the work orientation and burn-out of teachers.* Unpublished doctoral dissertation, University of California, Berkeley, 1979.

[11]Katz, M., & Zimbardo, P. G. Making it as a mental patient. *Psychology Today,* 1977, *10*(11), 122-126.

[12]Jones, J. What the kids taught the substitute. *San Francisco Chronicle,* February 20, 1979. © San Francisco Chronicle, 1979. Reprinted by permission of James M. Jones.

[13]Jackman, N., Schottstaedt, W., McPhail, S. C., & Wolf, S. Interaction, emotion, and physiologic change. *Journal of Health and Human Behavior,* 1963, *4,* 83-87. Reprinted by permission of the American Sociological Association and the authors.

[14]Torchia, J. Where crises are a way of life. *San Francisco Chronicle,* November 25, 1977. © San Francisco Chronicle, 1977. Reprinted by permission.

[15]Steiner, C. M. *Scripts people live.* New York: Grove Press, 1974. © 1974 by Claude Steiner. Reprinted by permission of Grove Press, Inc. and Bantam Books, Inc.

[16] Reprinted with permission of the publisher and the author, Dr. Philip Alper from *California Living Magazine* of the *San Francisco Sunday Examiner and Chronicle*, Copyright © 1976, San Francisco Examiner.

[17] Sager, C. J., & Hunt, B. *Intimate partners: Hidden patterns in love relationships.* New York: McGraw-Hill, 1979. Used by permission of the publisher.

[18] *Academe,* December 1978. © 1978 by the American Association of University Professors. Reprinted by permission of the publisher and the author.

[19] *Aged patients in long-term care facilities.* U.S. Department of Health, Education and Welfare, DHEW Publication No. (ADM) 76-154. Washington, D.C.: U.S. Government Printing Office, 1973.

CHAPTER 3–THE JOB SETTING AS A SOURCE OF BURNOUT

[1] Burnt-out principals. *Newsweek,* March 13, 1978. Copyright © 1978, by Newsweek, Inc. All rights reserved. Reprinted by permission.

[2] Robin Cook, The new doctor's dilemma. *Newsweek,* May 14, 1973. © 1973, by Newsweek, Inc. All rights reserved. Reprinted by permission of the author.

[3] Hughes, E. C. *The sociological eye: Selected papers.* Chicago: Aldine, 1971.

[4] Maslach, C., Jackson, S. E., & Barad, C. B. *Patterns of burnout among a national sample of public contact workers.* Unpublished manuscript, 1982.

[5] Maslach, C., & Pines, A. The burn-out syndrome in the day care setting. *Child Care Quarterly,* 1977, *6,* 100-113.

[6] Reprinted with permission of the publisher and the author, Nick Kazan, from *California Living Magazine* of the *San Francisco Examiner and Chronicle,* Copyright © 1972, San Francisco Examiner.

[7] Maslach, C., & Jackson, S. E. Lawyer burn-out. *Barrister,* 1978, *5*(2), 8; 52-54. Reprinted by permission of the publisher.

[8] Bramhall, M., & Ezell, S. How burned out are you? *Public Welfare,* 1981, *39*(1), 23-27. © 1981 American Public Welfare Association. Reprinted by permission of the publisher and the author.

[9] Terkel, S. *Working.* New York: Pantheon Books, 1974. © 1972, 1974 by Studs Terkel. Reprinted with permission of Pantheon Books, a Division of Random House, Inc.

[10] Van Hoose, W. H. Conflicts in counselor preparation and professional practice: An analysis. *Counselor Education and Supervision,* 1970, *9*(4), 241-247. Used by permission of the publisher.

[11] *Human Rights,* Summer 1978, 7(2), 6. Used by permission of the publisher.

[12] From *The sane society* by Erich Fromm. Copyright © 1955 by Erich Fromm. Reprinted by permission of Holt, Rinehart and Winston, Publishers.

[13] Armstrong, K. L. *An exploratory study of the interrelationships between worker characteristics, organizational structure, management process, and worker alienation from clients.* Unpublished doctoral dissertation, University of California, Berkeley, 1977.

[14] By Betty Harris, October 1976, *Sound Tracts,* 2(2). Reprinted by permission of the author and of the editor of *Sound Tracts,* Ron Curtis, Experience Education, Red Oak, Iowas.

CHAPTER 4—PERSONAL CHARACTERISTICS AS A SOURCE OF BURNOUT

[1] Gann, M.L. *The role of personality factors and job characteristics in burnout: A study of social service workers.* Unpublished doctoral dissertation, University of California, Berkeley, 1979. Used by permission of the author.

[2] Hall, R. C. W., Gardner, E. R., Perl, M., Stickney, S., & Pfefferbaum, B. The professional burnout syndrome. *Psychiatric Opinion,* 1979, *16*(4), 12-17. © 1979 by Opinion Publications, Inc. and reprinted by permission of the authors.

[3] Maslach, C., & Jackson, S. E. *The Maslach Burnout Inventory.* (Research ed.). Palo Alto, Calif.: Consulting Psychologists Press, 1981.

[4] Maslach, C., Jackson, S. E., & Barad, C. B. *Patterns of burnout among a national sample of public contact workers.* Unpublished manuscript, 1982.

[5] Gann, M. L. *The role of personality factors and job characteristics in burnout: A study of social service workers.* Unpublished doctoral dissertation, University of California, Berkeley, 1979. Heckman, S. J. *Effects of work setting, theoretical orientation, and personality on psychotherapist burnout.* Unpublished doctoral dissertation, California School of Professional Psychology, Berkeley, 1980.

[6] Bittker, T. E. Reaching out to the depressed physician. *Journal of the American Medical Association,* 1976, *236*(15), 1713-16. Copyright © 1976, American Medical Association. Reprinted by permission of the publisher and the author.

[7] Freudenberger, H. J. The staff burn-out syndrome in alternative institutions. *Psychotherapy: Theory, Research, and Practice,* 1975, *12*(1), 73-82. Reprinted by permission of the publisher.

[8] Saxon, S., & Kramer, A. L. *Suicide prevention center volunteers: An interpersonal perspective.* Paper presented at the annual convention of the Western Psychological Association, Sacramento, April 1975. Used by permission.

[9] Fromm-Reichmann, F. Notes on the personal and professional requirements of a psychotherapist. *Psychiatry,* 1949, *12*(14), 361-378.

[10] Letter appearing in the Ann Landers column of the *San Francisco Examiner,* April 19, 1981. © 1981 Field Newspaper Syndicate and reprinted with permission of Ann Landers.

[11] Lifton, R. J. The concept of the survivor. In J. E. Dimsdale (Ed.), *Survivors, victims, and perpetrators.* New York: Hemisphere, 1980.

CHAPTER 5—THE EFFECTS OF BURNOUT

[1] Adapted from material presented in Bennett-Sandler, G., & Ubell, E. Time bombs in blue. *New York Magazine,* March 21, 1977. Copyright © 1977 by News Group Publication, Inc. Reprinted with the permission of *New York Magazine.*

[2] What happens when nurses hit the bottle? by Judy Klemersrud. Copyright © 1978 by The New York Times Company. Reprinted by permission.

[3]Freudenberger, H. J. The staff burn-out syndrome in alternative institutions. *Psychotherapy: Theory, Research, and Practice,* 1975, *12*(1), 73-82.

[4]Ibid.

[5]Bittker, T. E. Reaching out to the depressed physician. *Journal of the American Medical Association,* 1976, *236*(15), 1713-16. Copyright © 1976, American Medical Association.

[6]John W. Goppelt, M.D. Letter to the editor, *Journal of the American Medical Association,* 1978, *239*(6), 495. Copyright © 1978, American Medical Association. Used by permission of the publisher and the author.

[7]Sheppe, W. M., Jr., & Stevenson, I. Techniques of interviewing. In H. I. Lief, V. F. Lief, & N. R. Lief (Eds.), *The psychology basis of medical practice.* New York: Lippincott/Harper & Row, 1963. Used by permission of the publisher.

[8]Maslach, C., Jackson, S. E., & Barad, C. B. *Patterns of burnout among a national sample of public contact workers.* Unpublished manuscript, 1982.

[9]Thorne, F. C. Games psychologists play. *Journal of Community Psychology,* 1975, *3,* 175-181. Used by permission of the publisher.

[10]Adapted from Maslach, C., & Jackson, S. E. Burned-out cops and their families. *Psychology Today,* 1979, *12*(12), 59-62. Copyright © 1979 by Ziff-Davis Publishing Company.

CHAPTER 6–HOW TO HANDLE BURNOUT: DOING IT ON YOUR OWN

[1]Koocher, G. P. Pediatric cancer: Psychosocial problems and the high costs of helping. *Journal of Clinical Child Psychology,* 1980, *10,* 2-5. Used by permission of the publisher.

[2]Jones, J. What the kids taught the substitute. *San Francisco Chronicle,* February 20, 1979. © San Francisco Chronicle, 1979. Reprinted by permission of James M. Jones.

[3]In my earliest writing on burnout, I used the term *time-out* for this type of work change, since that was the word used by several caregivers in their interviews with me. However, that particular term has led to erroneous interpretations, since it is more suggestive of a work *break* (calling a halt to work in order to rest) rather than a work *change* (shifting from one task to a less demanding one). Because of this conceptual confusion, I am now calling this technique a "downshift" instead of a "time-out."

[4]Elrod, S. Job burnout: What to do if your job isn't fun anymore. *St. Paul Dispatch.* Used by permission of the publisher.

[5]Koocher, G. P. Adjustment and coping strategies among the caretakers of cancer patients. Reprinted from *Social Work in Health Care,* 1979, *5*(2), 145-150. © 1979 by The Haworth Press, Inc. Used by permission. All rights reserved.

[6]Heckman, S. J. *Effects of work setting, theoretical orientation, and personality on psychotherapist burnout.* Unpublished doctoral dissertation, California School of Professional Psychology, Berkeley, 1980.

[7]Adapted from *The American way of life need not be hazardous to your health* by John W. Farquhar, M.D., by permission of the author and W. W. Norton & Company, Inc. Copyright © 1978 by John W. Farquhar. Originally published as part of the Portable Stanford, published by the Stanford Alumni Association, Stanford, California.

[8]Caplan, G. *Social support and community mental health.* New York: Basic Books, 1974.

Cobb, S. Social support as a moderator of life stress. *Psychosomatic Medicine,* 1976, *38,* 300-314.

Dean, A., & Lin, N. The stress-buffering role of social support: Problems and prospects for systematic investigation. *Journal of Nervous and Mental Disease,* 1977, *165,* 403-417.

Gottlieb, B. H. (Ed.), *Social networks and social support.* Beverly Hills, Calif.: Sage Publications, 1981.

[9]Maatz, L. How three tough cops found solace in Christ. *San Francisco Examiner,* March 11, 1979. Used by permission of the publisher.

CHAPTER 7—HOW TO HANDLE BURNOUT: SOCIAL AND ORGANIZATIONAL APPROACHES

[1]Carol Hutelmyer, RN, MSN, Director of Nurses, Thomas Jefferson University School of Nursing, Philadelphia. Quoted in Shubin, S. Burnout: The professional hazard you face in nursing. *Nursing78,* 1978, *8*(7), 22-27. Reprinted with permission from the July issue of *Nursing78.* Copyright © 1978 Intermed Communications, Inc.

[2]Long, N., & Newman, R. G. The teacher and his mental health. *The Teacher's Handling of Children in Conflict,* Bulletin of School of Education, Indiana University, July 1961, pp. 5-26. Used by permission of the publisher.

[3]Koocher, G. P. Adjustment and coping strategies among the caretakers of cancer patients. *Social Work in Health Care,* 1979, *5*(2), 145-150.

[4]Freudenberger, H. J. The staff burn-out syndrome in alternative institutions. *Psychotherapy: Theory, Research, and Practice,* 1975, *12*(1), 73-82.

[5]Freudenberger, H. J. *The staff burn-out syndrome.* Washington, D.C.: Drug Abuse Council, 1975. Reprinted by permission of the author.

[6]Pines, A., & Maslach, C. Combatting staff burnout in a day care center: A case study. *Child Care Quarterly,* 1980, *9,* 5-16.

[7]Seligman, M. E. P. *Helplessness: On depression, development, and death.* San Francisco: W. H. Freeman, 1975.

[8]Langer, E., & Rodin, J. The effects of choice and enhanced personal responsibility for the aged: A field experiment in an institutional setting. *Journal of Personality and Social Psychology,* 1976, *34,* 191-198.

Rodin, J., & Langer, E. Long-term effects of a control-relevant intervention with the institutionalized aged. *Journal of Personality and Social Psychology,* 1977, *35,* 897-902.

CHAPTER 8—PREVENTING BURNOUT

[1]Savicki, V. *An approach to conceptualizing, treating, and preventing burnout.* Paper presented at the Oregon Psychological Association Fall Conference, October 1979. Used by permission.

[2]Miller, H. S., Jr. Is the bedside manner a terminal case? *Harvard Magazine,* July-August 1979. Copyright © 1979 Harvard Magazine. Reprinted by permission.

[3] Maslach, C., & Pines, A. The burn-out syndrome in the day care setting. *Child Care Quarterly*, 1977, *6*, 100-113.

[4] Pines, A., & Maslach, C. Combatting staff burnout in a day care center: A case study. *Child Care Quarterly*, 1980, *9*, 5-16.

[5] Maslach, C., & Jackson, S. E. *The Maslach Burnout Inventory*. (Research Ed.). Palo Alto, Calif.: Consulting Psychologists Press, 1981.

[6] Moos, R. H. *The social climate scales*. Palo Alto, Calif.: Consulting Psychologists Press, 1974.

[7] Miles, M. B., Hornstein, H. A., Calder, P. H., Callahan, D. M., & Schiavo, R. S. Data feedback: A rationale. In H. A. Hornstein, B. B. Bunker, W. W. Burke, M. Gindes, & R. J. Lewicki (Eds.), *Social intervention: A behavioral science approach*. New York: Free Press, 1971.

[8] Maslach, C., & Jackson, S. E. Lawyer burn-out. *Barrister*, 1978, *5*(2), 8; 52-54.

[9] Storlie, F. J. Burnout: The elaboration of a concept. *American Journal of Nursing*, 1979, *19*(12), 2108-11. Used by permission.

[10] Wanous, J. P. Organizational entry: Newcomers moving from outside to inside. *Psychological Bulletin*, 1977, *84*, 601-618.

[11] Examples of such books are: Shulman, L. *The skills of helping individuals and groups*. Itasca, Ill.: F. E. Peacock Publishers, 1979. Berger, M. M. *Working with people called patients*. New York: Brunner/Mazel, 1977.

[12] Danish, S. J., & Hauer, A. L. *Helping skills: A basic training program*. New York: Behavioral Publications, 1973.

[13] Werner, E. R., Adler, R., Robinson, R., & Korsch, B. M. Attitudes and interpersonal skills during pediatric internship. *Pediatrics*, 1979, *63*(2), 491-499. Copyright © 1979, American Academy of Pediatrics. Reprinted by permission of the publisher.

[14] Maluccio, A. N. *Learning from clients*. New York: Free Press, 1979.

[15] P.L.U.M. Community Connection. Project Director: Norma Jean Orlando. Elgin Mental Health Center, 750 S. State Street, Elgin, Illinois 60120.

[16] Benarde, M. A., & Mayerson, E. W. Patient-physician negotiation. *Journal of the American Medical Association*, 1978, 239(14), 1413-15. Copyright © 1978, American Medical Association. Used by permission of the publisher and the author.

APPENDIX—TECHNIQUES FOR STRESS MANAGEMENT

[1] Reprinted from *The American way of life need not be hazardous to your health* by John W. Farquhar, M.D., by permission of the author and W. W. Norton & Company, Inc. Copyright © 1978 by John W. Farquhar. Originally published by the Stanford Alumni Association, Stanford, California.

BIBLIOGRAPHY

ARTICLES AND CHAPTERS

Alexander, C. J. Counteracting burnout. *American Operating Room Nurses (AORN) Journal,* 1980, *32,* 597-604. Gives description of burnout syndrome and discusses possible causes at both personal and organizational levels. Suggests a variety of coping techniques. (10 refs.)

Alexander, R. J. "Burning out" versus "punching out." *Journal of Human Stress,* 1980, *6*(1), 37-41. Presents three case histories of "burnout" in air traffic controllers. Their burnout is characterized by depression, anxiety, fear of midair collision, insomnia, and lack of confidence in job capabilities. Burned-out controllers are retired and then symptoms decrease or disappear, but the controllers report little or no desire to return to work. (Note that the concept of *burnout* used here is not the same as burnout for helping professionals.) (8 refs.)

Austin, D. A. Renewal. *Journal of Physical Education and Recreation,* 1980, *51*(9), 57-59. Focuses on the importance of inservice programs dealing with motivation and job satisfaction of physical education teachers. Offers several suggestions for preventing burnout. Encourages professional growth enhancement through membership in national physical education associations. Preceded by checklist of 79 suggestions for preventing burnout (pp. 53-54) and followed by case history of support group of physical education teachers (p. 60). (2 refs.)

Bardo, P. The pain of teacher burnout: A case history. *Phi Delta Kappan,* 1979, *61*(4), 252-254. Presents one person's account of burning out as a teacher and starting over as a stockbroker. Discusses the deterioration in student interest and participation as a major cause of teacher burnout. Proposes that the fundamental problem that is destroying schools and demoralizing teachers is a devaluation of education.

Boy, A. V., & Pine, G. J. Avoiding counselor burnout through role renewal. *Personnel and Guidance Journal,* 1980, *59,* 161-163. Emphasizes the need for counselors to reassess their role as counselors and to recommit themselves to counseling. Major focus is on the individual's responsibility to counseling. Recommends counselors focus on clients' needs, establish relationships with committed colleagues, become involved with their organizations, and dedicate themselves to a particular theoretical approach. (16 refs.)

Bramhall, M., & Ezell, S. How burned out are you? *Public Welfare,* 1981, *39*(1), 23-27. First of a three-part series on burnout. Distinguishes burnout from depression. Uses a model developed by stress researcher Hans Selye to demonstrate how human service workers burn out. Offers a test that indicates "your danger of burning out": ten questions in each of the following categories (job, attitude, feelings, behavior). (8 refs.)

Bramhall, M., & Ezell, S. Working your way out of burnout. *Public Welfare,* 1981, *39*(2), 32-39. Second of a three-part series on burnout. Emphasizes a personal regimen for treating burnout that enables the individual to exercise detached concern. Treatment plan was developed through work with hundreds of professionals and is a four-week regimen that includes cutting back on work load, getting rest and exercise, and having a proper diet. (6 refs.)

Bramhall, M., & Ezell, S. How agencies can prevent burnout. *Public Welfare,* 1981, *39*(3), 33-37. Third of a three-part series on burnout. Offers suggestions for system management for prevention of burnout. Emphasizes role of the immediate supervisor as a burnout "troubleshooter." Suggests "buddy system" as important for prevention and encourages organizations to establish training in stress management, time management, and self-care. Gives thirteen suggestions for preventing burnout. (10 refs.)

Brockman, N. Burnout in superiors. *Review for Religious,* 1978, *37,* 809-816. Discusses the following contributions to burnout in religious superiors: (a) built-in frustration of inheriting seemingly insurmountable long-term questions; (b) lack of good personnel; (c) economics; (d) lack of colleagueship; (e) working with people who are disillusioned with religion; (f) distance from ideas, fresh insights, or broader views of reality; and (g) sense of responsibility for problems that cannot be resolved due to a lack of resources. Presents coping strategies.

Bundy, O. K. Everything you always wanted to know about professional burnout but were afraid to ask. *Contemporary Education,* 1981, *53*(1), 9-11. Gives a brief summary of burnout symptoms. Discusses burnout as it affects teachers and counselors, and concludes that the main cause of burnout is stress. (10 refs.)

Cardinell, C. F. Burnout? Mid-life Crisis? Let's understand ourselves. *Contemporary Education,* 1981, *52*(2), 103-108. Proposes that stress, career burnout, and mid-life professional crisis are related stages in career development. States that emphasis should be placed on understanding causes rather than cures. Analyzes causes by reviewing research on Maslow's theory of human motivation. Concludes that the most hazardous time for burnout is when commitment to professional ideals outstrips satisfaction from life and work. Recommends more awareness of the dynamics of professional maturation, clear definitions of terms for research purposes, and longitudinal research on professional development. (21 refs.)

Carroll, J. F. X. Staff burnout as a form of ecological dysfunction. *Contemporary Drug Problems,* 1980, *8,* 207-225. Concise overview of burnout. Stresses the interactional nature of burnout. Outlines physical, psychological, social and systems burnout symptoms. Discusses treatment directed at individuals, at work environments, and at nonwork ecosystems. Means of prevention are also outlined. (14 refs.)

Chamberlin, C. S. Anomie, burnout and the Wyatt Earp syndrome. *Law and Order,* March 1978, *26,* 20-21, 52. Discusses burnout among police officers and proposes several hypotheses about which officers will be more at risk. Suggests several ways of dealing with burnout. (5 refs.)

Cherniss, C., Egnatios, E. S., Wacker, S., & O'Dowd, B. The professional mystique and burnout in public sector professionals. *Social Policy,* in press. Proposes that the major cause of burnout in professionals working in the public sector is "professional mystique," which includes beliefs that: (a) professionals have autonomy in their work; (b) professional work is always interesting; (c) credentials automatically mean competence; (d) collegial relationships are always strong and supportive; (e) clients are always cooperative and grateful; (f) professionals are always sympathetic and compassionate. Argues that mystique leads to unrealistic expectations and disillusionment, and contributes to lack of concern about personnel policies and job structure in the institutions. Discusses implications for social policy, with emphasis on realistic training, recruitment, and selection procedures. (22 refs.)

Christensen, J. Burning and burnout. *English Journal,* 1981, *70*(4), 13-16. Discusses burnout as it relates to the teaching profession. Explores the meanings of the metaphors "burning" and "burnout" as they relate to the work and lives of teachers. Provides suggestions for "tending the fire."

Collins, G. R. Burnout: The hazard of professional helpers. *Christianity Today,* 1977, *21*(13), 12-14. Relates the basic symptoms and remedies of burnout to Christian helpers. Suggests frequent prayer and meditation as remedies for burnout.

Daley, M. R. Burnout: Smoldering problem in protective services. *Social Work,* 1979, *24,* 375-379. Gives general overview of burnout in social services. Within the specific area of child protective services, proposes that agencies tacitly encourage turnover among workers by failing to devise career ladders in direct services. Inability to advance in careers may lead to lack of incentive, which then contributes to burnout. (7 refs.)

Daley, M. R. Preventing worker burnout in child welfare. *Child Welfare*, 1979, *58*(7), 443-450. Discusses factors that contribute to and that inhibit burnout. Brings together many research findings and relates them to personal and organizational aspects of child welfare work. (11 refs.)

Daniel, S., & Rogers, S. L. Burnout and the pastorate: A critical review with implications for pastors. *Journal of Psychology and Theology*, 1981, *9*(3), 232-249. Scholarly review of burnout literature divided into the following categories: anecdotal, theoretical, experimental, prescriptive. Within each category literature is further delineated in terms of whether it covers intrapersonal and/or systems variables of burnout. Discusses aspects of ministry that lead to burnout and offers recommendations for prevention for the individual, the church, and the denomination. (52 refs.)

Ellison, K. W., & Genz, J. L. The police officer as burned-out Samaritan. *FBI Law Enforcement Bulletin*, 1978, *47*(3), 1-7. Discusses aspects of police work that contribute to burnout. Says patrol officers who must deal with too many cases that demand contradictory skills are particularly vulnerable. Considers causes of extreme stress to be the wounding or killing of a fellow officer and cases that involve child abuse. Cites the "military model" of police work as a major organizational contributor to burnout. Discusses need for "ventilation" of officers' feelings and outlines methods of coping. (11 refs.)

Emener, W. G., Jr. Professional burnout: Rehabilitation's hidden handicap. *Journal of Rehabilitation*, 1979, *45*(1), 55-58. Discusses the symptoms of professional burnout and identifies situational conditions unique to the field of rehabilitation that contribute to professional burnout. Suggests preventative strategies and offers suggestions for helping the burnout candidate. (11 refs.)

Foster, R. E. Burnout among teachers of severely handicapped, autistic children. *Pointer*, 1980, *24*(2), 24-28. Discusses stages experienced by teachers of autistic children: survival, transition, creativity, burnout. Outlines burnout traps: confusing the easy way with efficiency, unimaginative use of time, repetition of curriculum, insulation from outside ideas, inability to ask for help, trying harder rather than more intelligently, measuring oneself solely by children's accomplishments (or lack of them). Offers three points for personal growth. (3 refs.)

Freudenberger, H. J. Staff burn-out. *Journal of Social Issues*, 1974, *30*(1), 159-165. Discusses both physical and behavioral signs of burnout. Describes the burnout-prone individual as one who is dedicated and committed, and/or one who gets bogged down in the routinization of the job. Outlines ten preventative measures and offers suggestions for helping the burnout victim. (3 refs.)

Freudenberger, H. J. The staff burn-out syndrome in alternative institutions. *Psychotherapy: Theory, Research, and Practice*, 1975, *12*(1), 73-82. Discusses the following personality types as burnout prone: (a) dedicated, committed workers who are caught between their own needs, their clients' needs, and the administrators' needs; (b) overcommitted staff members whose outside life is subsatisfactory; (c) authoritarians who do not believe anyone else can do the job as well as they can; (d) overworked administrators; (e) professionals who lend their services to an alternative institution.

Discusses symptoms, preventative measures, and suggestions for help that were first presented in Freudenberger (1974). (6 refs.)

Freudenberger, H. J. Burn-out: Occupational hazard of the child care worker. *Child Care Quarterly*, 1977, *56*, 90-99. Describes symptoms of burnout and discusses the following job stresses that may lead to burnout: decision making without adequate time, taking work problems home, lack of opportunity to see progress with children, inadequate decision-making training, lack of communication among staff. Suggestions for individuals and agencies are offered. (4 refs.)

Freudenberger, H. J. Burn-out: The organizational menace. *Training and Development Journal*, 1977, *31*(7), 26-27. Outlines symptoms of burnout within an organizational setting. Suggests an indirect approach to helping someone who is burned out because the direct approach may be met with defensive resistance.

Friel, M., & Tehan, C. Counteracting burn-out for the hospice caregiver. *Cancer Nursing*, 1980, *3*(4), 285-293. Describes burnout in the context of hospice home care. Discusses sources of stress, including: (a) the nature of terminal illness; (b) the physical and emotional demands of the work; (c) resistance from other medical staff; (d) exaggerated expectations of the caregiver; (e) emotional involvement with patients and families; (f) clash between ideals and reality. Offers suggestions for intervention in the areas of patient contact, interpersonal skills, social support systems, administration, and personal coping techniques. (11 refs.)

Garfield, C. A. Coping with burn-out. *Hospital Forum*, 1980, *23*, 15. Brief description of burnout among health professionals. Lists behavior changes that accompany burnout and situations that contribute to it. Lists six individual antidotes and six group antidotes for burnout.

Garte, S. H., & Rosenblum, M. L. Lighting fires in burned-out counselors. *Personnel and Guidance Journal.* 1978, *57*, 158-160. Describes the development of and provides examples of workshop exercises designed to bring together work and leisure for counselors. Proposes that the fusion of work and leisure will help the counselor "recharge" and thus not burn out. (7 refs.)

Gill, J. J. Burnout: A growing threat in ministry. *Human Development*, 1980, *1*(2), 21-27. Reviews and summarizes findings by burnout researchers. Gives overview of burnout symptoms and causes. Discusses 11 types of religious people who may be most vulnerable to burnout. (6 refs.)

Ginsberg, S. G. The problem of the burned out executive. *Personnel Journal*, 1974, *53*, 598-600. Brief general discussion of burnout among executives. Offers ten suggestions for combating burnout.

Golembiewski, R. T., & Munzenrider, R. Efficacy of three versions of one burnout measure: The MBI as total score, sub-scale scores, or phases? *Journal of Health and Human Resources Administration*, 1981, *4*, 228-246. Analyzes the merits of three different ways of scoring the Maslach Burnout Inventory (MBI). Presents research findings on the correlations between the MBI and several variables in the work setting. Provides supportive evidence for the usefulness of all three versions of the MBI, but argues that the phase model may prove to be the best approach to understanding burnout. (20 refs.)

Hall, R. C. W., Gardner, E. R., Perl, M., Stickney, S. K., & Pfefferbaum, B. The professional burnout syndrome. *Psychiatric Opinion*, 1979, *16*(4), 12-17. Defines the etiology and symptoms of burnout as it occurs in health care settings and explores some of the social forces that produce burnout. Outlines six physical symptoms and seven behavioral symptoms. Cites a case study of individual burnout. Gives ten symptoms of organizational burnout, and offers ten suggestions to management for the prevention of burnout. (3 refs.)

Harrison, D. Role strain and burnout in child protective service workers. *Social Service Review*, 1980, *54*, 31-44. Reports results of survey research of 112 child protective service workers. Findings show that workers experienced a high degree of role conflict and role ambiguity, which was correlated with work dissatisfaction. Suggests that workers need to be clear about what is expected of them in fulfilling their role in order to feel good about their work. (13 refs.)

Hendrickson, B. Teacher burnout: How to recognize it; what to do about it. *Learning*, 1979, *7*, 36-39. Gives anecdotes about teacher burnout and about teachers who are successfully combating this syndrome. Offers seventeen suggestions for fighting burnout.

Jackson, S. E., & Maslach, C. After-effects of job-related stress: Families as victims. *Journal of Occupational Behaviour*, 1982, *3*, 63-77. Reports on research in which 142 police officers and their wives described family interactions and officers were administered the Maslach Burnout Inventory (MBI). Officers who were experiencing burnout were more likely to display anger, to spend time away from home, to be uninvolved with concerns of family life, and to have unhappy marriages. Suggests how police administrators might help their officers cope with job stress and lessen its detrimental impact on police families. (28 refs.)

Jones, J. W. Dishonesty, burnout, and unauthorized work break extensions. *Personality and Social Psychology Bulletin*, 1981, *7*(3), 406-409. Reports on survey research with thirty-one nurses who completed a dishonesty scale, a burnout scale, and a behavioral checklist that measured how often they took unauthorized extensions of work and food breaks. Burned-out nurses extended their work breaks more often than did non-burned-out nurses. Burnout scores predicted work break (but not food break) extensions. (19 refs.)

Jones, M. A., & Emanuel, J. There is life after burnout. *The High School Journal*, 1981, *64*, 209-212. Describes burnout in the teaching profession and proposes a three-stage model: Heating Up, Boiling, and Explosion. Discusses a corresponding three-stage model of recovery from burnout, in which each stage has a threefold focus on self, environment, and professional skills. (4 refs.)

Kahn, R. Job burnout: Prevention and remedies. *Public Welfare*, 1978, *36*(2), 61-63. Discusses related research and argues that the main cause of burnout is role conflict, and especially work overload. Offers the following burnout remedies: better selection and training, reduction in amount of direct client contact, and increased social support on the job.

Kammer, A. Burnout—contemporary dilemma for the Jesuit activist. *Studies in the Spirituality of Jesuits*, 1978, *10*(1), 1-20. Discusses many issues that contribute to burnout in Jesuits, with emphasis on the struggle between church and "real world" demands. Followed by replies from American, Mexican, and French Jesuits. (2 refs.)

Lamb, R. H. Staff burnout in work with long-term patients. *Hospital and Community Psychiatry,* 1979, *30,* 396-398. Discusses burnout in mental health professionals who work with severely disabled individuals. Burnout stems from unrealistic view of rehabilitation and the lack of an individualistic approach to clients' treatment. Misapplication of concept of normalization contributes to frustrations, as does administrative pressure on staff to produce impossible results. (7 refs.)

Lammert, M. A. A group experience to combat burnout and learn group process skills. *Journal of Nursing Education,* 1981, *20*(6), 41-46. Proposes a program for helping to prevent burnout by participating in and learning about group processes. Describes participation in program by four hundred undergraduates (half were juniors in a BA program and half were registered nurses returning to school for their BSN). Program placed major emphasis on becoming more self-aware and learning how to develop and maintain collaborative relationships. Presents this program as particularly useful to nurses who must work with a variety of people. (13 refs.)

Larson, C. C., Gilbertson, D. L., & Powell, J. A. Therapist burnout: Perspectives on a critical issue. *Social Casework,* 1978, *59,* 563-565. Briefly examines causes and remedies for therapist burnout. Proposes that the major contributing factor is constant pressure to meet emotional needs and desires of clients and remain "selfless" while doing so. Suggests that burnout be avoided through restructuring of mental health attitudes and environment in a way that will incorporate concern for therapist differentiation and nurturance.

Lattanzi, M. E. Coping with work-related losses. *Personnel and Guidance Journal,* 1981, *59,* 350-351. Briefly discusses the way hospices are structured, using an interdisciplinary team approach that provides a network of mutual support and learning. This approach aids in burnout prevention and is recommended for any organization whose staff are involved in emotionally draining work.

Lewiston, N. J., Conley, J., & Blessing-Moore, J. Measurement of hypothetical burnout in cystic fibrosis caregivers. *Acta Paediatrica Scandinavica,* 1981, *70,* 935-939. Reports on research using the Maslach Burnout Inventory (MBI) with ninety-six health professionals attending workshops. Results showed that emotional exhaustion was higher for cystic fibrosis caregivers than for professionals in other areas of specialty pediatrics. Within the cystic fibrosis group, those who spent a greater percentage of their time with sick, hospitalized patients had higher burnout scores. (17 refs.)

MacNiece, J. Burnout. *Women's Work,* 1979, *5*(5), 5-10; 27. Relates burnout to "women's work" and the stresses it involves. Calls for organization on all levels. Offers one-page anecdote of one woman's burnout experience.

Marshall, R. E., & Kasman, C. Burnout in the neonatal intensive care unit. *Pediatrics,* 1980, *65,* 1161-65. Defines burnout as the loss of motivation for creative involvement and discusses it in terms of health professionals working in a neonatal intensive care unit. Presents characteristics and causes of burnout from a clinical perspective. Offers strategies for reducing and coping with burnout. (16 refs.)

Maslach, C. Burned-out. *Human Behavior,* 1976, *5*(9), 16-22. Summarizes the major findings from studies with 200 professionals in health and social services. Discusses the following correlates of burnout: cynicism, reference to clients in derogatory or abstract terms, rigid adherence to rules, extreme detachment, psychosomatic illnesses, and family problems. Discusses the following systems contributions to burnout: heavy case load, little or no emotional support, no "time-out" periods, long hours of continuous client contact, inadequate training. Offers recommendations for dealing with burnout.

Maslach, C. The client role in staff burnout. *Journal of Social Issues,* 1978, *34*(4), 111-124. Analyzes the following client factors as important contributors to staff burnout: the type and severity of clients' problems, the prognosis of change or cure, the degree of personal relevance of the clients' problems for the staff member, the rules governing staff-client interaction, the clients' reactions to staff. Suggests that steps to humanize the staff-client relationship must focus on both participants in the interaction. (11 refs.)

Maslach, C. Job burnout: How people cope. *Public Welfare,* 1978, *36*(2), 56-58. Discusses burnout in terms of the emotional exhaustion resulting from the stress of interpersonal contact. Summarizes findings from research on helping professionals. Discusses techniques of psychological withdrawal that these professionals use.

Maslach, C. The burn-out syndrome and patient care. In C. A. Garfield (Ed.), *Stress and survival: The emotional realities of life-threatening illness.* St. Louis: Mosby, 1979. Discusses the experience of burnout for health professionals, with special emphasis on the emotional strains of caring for dying patients. Suggests various prevention and coping techniques: training in interpersonal skills, analysis of personal feelings, social-professional support system, use of humor, amount and variety of patient contact, separation between work and home (and use of decompression activities), and physical health. (13 refs.)

Maslach, C. Burnout: A social psychological analysis. In J. W. Jones (Ed.), *The burnout syndrome: Current research, theory, interventions.* Park Ridge, Ill.: London House Press, 1981. A theoretical analysis of the burnout syndrome from the perspective of social psychology. Key themes include: biases in the attribution process, factors that promote a negative and dehumanized perception of recipients, and the role of other people in various coping strategies. Findings on situational factors in burnout and on individual detachment techniques are also summarized. (29 refs.)

Maslach, C. Understanding burnout: Definitional issues in analyzing a complex phenomenon. In W. S. Paine (Ed.), *Job stress and Burnout.* Beverly Hills, Ca.: Sage Publications, 1982. Discusses problems in defining burnout and the implications for theory, research, and application. Analyzes common elements of these definitions and changes in the development of the concept. Points to promising trends in future work on burnout. (20 refs.)

Maslach, C., & Jackson, S. E. Lawyer burnout. *Barrister,* 1978, *5*(2), 8; 52-54. Studies with lawyers show that the combination of excessive case load and lack of challenging and prestigious test cases and law reform work could be contributing factors to burnout. The goals and expectations of legal services attorneys often do not coincide with the realities of the job. Suggestions for preventing burnout include the development of interviewing and counseling skills.

Maslach, C., & Jackson, S. E. Burned-out cops and their families. *Psychology Today*, 1979, *12*(12), 59-62. Discusses research on 130 police families in which the Maslach Burnout Inventory (MBI) was completed by the officers and both they and their wives answered questions about their home life. High burnout scores were associated with domestic strains. Younger officers scored higher on burnout than older officers. Officers' emotional cool, suspiciousness, and caution were found to extend to family relationships. While 80 percent of the wives sought out organized activities as a source of help and social support, only 10 percent of the officers did so. (4 refs.)

Maslach, C., & Jackson, S. E. The measurement of experienced burnout. *Journal of Occupational Behaviour*, 1981, *2*, 99-113. Discusses the construction of the Maslach Burnout Inventory (MBI), a twenty-two-item measure of burnout among people workers. The MBI contains three subscales: emotional exhaustion, depersonalization, and personal accomplishment (reverse scoring). Various psychometric analyses show that the MBI has both high reliability and validity as a measure of burnout. (23 refs.)

Maslach, C., & Jackson, S. E. Burnout in health professions: A social psychological analysis. In G. Sanders & J. Suls (Eds.), *Social psychology of health and illness*. Hillsdale, N.J.: Lawrence Erlbaum, 1982. Theory and research about burnout among health professionals. Theoretical points are illustrated by research studies of 169 nurses and 43 physicians in which the Maslach Burnout Inventory (MBI) was used to assess burnout. Discussion focuses on critical elements of the work situation (dealing with people, success and failure, control and lack of control, ambiguity), biases in individual perception and attribution, and patterns of coping strategies (getting away from versus turning toward others). (76 refs.)

Maslach, C., & Pines, A. The burnout syndrome in the day care setting. *Child Care Quarterly*, 1977, *6*, 100-113. Reports on survey of eighty-three staff members of day-care centers. Results show that: (a) staff-child ratio had impact on staff's reactions to the job and to children, (b) long hours of direct contact with children were associated with stress and negative attitudes, (c) "time-out" periods helped prevent burnout, (d) regular staff meetings increased job satisfaction, (e) good work relationships were associated with job satisfaction. Offers suggestions for prevention and a review of literature on dehumanization. (22 refs.)

Maslach, C., & Pines, A. Burnout: The loss of human caring. In A. Pines & C. Maslach (Eds.), *Experiencing social psychology*. New York: Knopf, 1979. Discusses and elaborates on summary findings presented in Maslach (1976). Analyzes detachment techniques and suggests remedies for burnout.

Mattingly, M. A. Sources of stress and burn-out in professional child care work. *Child Care Quarterly*, 1977, *6*, 127-137. Examines stress-producing aspects of clinical child care. Proposes that child-care workers' associations can help with problems of stress and burnout by making workers more aware of the sources of stress and the possibility of burnout, facilitating strong supportive relationships among members, and influencing training curricula so that professionals get a wider range of skills that can be used with various programs and types of children. (9 refs.)

McConnel, E. A. How close are you to burnout? *RN,* May 1981, *44*(5), 29-33. Describes burnout as the product of constant emotional stress over time, combinations of stressors, and individual ability to cope. Outlines characteristics and behaviors of patients and colleagues that contribute to frustration in nurses. Discusses list of stress factors in the health care environment, including shortage of personnel and shortage of supplies. Provides a "burnout worksheet" for assessment of physical, interpersonal, and behavioral symptoms in terms of their duration, frequency, and intensity. Offers 12 coping strategies. Followed by personal account of one nurse's burnout experience and recovery.

McGuire, W. H. Teacher burnout. *Today's Education*, 1979, *68*(4), 5. Editorial by the president of the National Education Association (NEA). Discusses violence and vandalism as two major contributors to the increase in teacher burnout. Gives statistics gathered in nationwide NEA Teacher Opinion Poll.

Meadow, K. P. Burnout in professionals working with deaf children. *American Annals of the Deaf,* 1981, *126*(1), 13-22. Reports on research using the Maslach Burnout Inventory (MBI) with 240 educators of deaf children. Emotional exhaustion was linked to the following factors: age, number of years working in the field, type of work, type of school, lack of job satisfaction, and lack of sense of power in work situation. Emotional exhaustion was higher for educators of deaf children than for teachers of nondisabled students. (11 refs.)

Moe, D. A. A prescription (for burnout). *Today's Education,* 1979, *68*(4), 35-36. Proposes sixteen suggestions for preventing burnout (based on the author's personal experiences).

Neville, S. H. Job stress and burnout: Occupational hazards for services staff. *College and Research Libraries,* 1981, *42,* 242-247. Discusses stress factors that may contribute to burnout in library staff members responsible for service delivery in academic libraries. Considers three components of job stress: (a) individual ability to handle stressful occupation, (b) traditional organizational structure, and (c) fragmented professional support. Discusses solutions in terms of productive individual coping strategies, enhanced organizational design, and cohesive professional support. (18 refs.)

Patrick, P. K. S. Burnout: Job hazard for health workers. *Hospitals,* 1979, *53*(22), 87-88; 90. Briefly outlines signs of burnout, including reduction in flexibility. Discusses both self-causes of burnout (lack of self-awareness and self-imposed restrictions) and system causes (stressful work and lack of system support for employees). Gives eight suggestions for burnout prevention.

Perlman, B., & Hartman, E. A. An integration of burnout into a stress model. ERIC-CAPS, 1980. Scholarly review of burnout research that integrates the burnout literature with stress research. Proposes that antecedents, prevention, and containment of burnout are best understood when placed in the context of a stress perspective. Discusses both theoretical and empirical work on burnout and stress and summarizes points of agreement. (46 refs.)

Perlman, B., & Hartman, E. A. Burnout: Summary and future research. *Human Relations,* in press. Summarizes burnout literature and provides analysis of definitions and research results. Presents model of burnout and suggests questions to be studied in future research. (73 refs.)

Pines, A. Burnout: A current problem in pediatrics. *Current Problems in Pediatrics,* 1981, *11*(7), 3-31. Draws on research findings and burnout workshops to discuss problems particular to pediatric workers. Discusses three burnout profiles in pediatric work: (a) the pediatrician whose work involves primary care of well children in outpatient settings where the main stresses are the routine and lack of challenge; (b) the pediatric nurse and doctor who work within the hospital setting and care for severely ill or dying children; (c) the pediatrician who works within an academic setting and must balance the demands of academia and of a medical practice. Discusses organizational contributors to burnout and outlines preventative measures. (38 refs.)

Pines, A. Helper's motivation and the burnout syndrome. In T. A. Wills (Ed.), *Basic processes in helping relationships.* New York: Academic Press, 1982. Defines burnout as physical, emotional, and mental exhaustion. Presents research findings and an analysis of the relationship between burnout and various work motivations. These motivations include those that are universally shared (money, significance, autonomy and growth, social networks), those that characterize helping professionals, and those that are unique to the individual helper. Discusses implications for training and for modification of the work environment. (43 refs.)

Pines, A., & Aronson, E. Combatting burnout. *Children and Youth Services Review,* in press. Describes study in which short- and long-term impact of a burnout workshop were evaluated. Fifty-three social service workers completed a questionnaire one week prior to the workshop. Some of them participated in the workshop, while the others did not. Questionnaires were administered again one week later, and participants showed slightly decreased burnout and greatly increased job satisfaction, while nonparticipants did not. Six-month follow-up revealed that the social aspects of the job had been improved by the workshop. (8 refs.)

Pines, A., & Kafry, D. Occupational tedium in the social services. *Social Work,* 1978, *23*(6), 499-507. Tedium is defined as the experience of physical, emotional, and attitudinal exhaustion and thus is related to burnout. Tedium was studied among 129 social service workers attending workshop on burnout. External aspects of work were correlated with tedium and work satisfaction; internal aspects of work were correlated with job satisfaction.

Pines, A., & Maslach, C. Characteristics of staff burn-out in mental health settings. *Hospital and Community Psychiatry,* 1978, *29,* 233-237. Reports results of survey study of seventy-six staff members in various mental health facilities. The longer staff had worked in the mental health field, the less they liked working with patients, the less successful they felt with them, and the less humanistic were their attitudes toward mental illness. Recommendations for reducing stress and burnout include allowing more chances for temporary withdrawal from direct patient care and changing the function of staff meetings to allow more open communication.

Pines, A., & Maslach, C. Combatting staff burn-out in a day care center: A case study. *Child Care Quarterly,* 1980, *9,* 5-16. Discusses intervention in a day-care center that changed the ratio of staff to children and gave more structure to the program. Results showed that children engaged in more constructive play, teachers had better interactions with children, and teachers felt more secure and less exhausted. Assesses the changes after six months and finds that they had mostly positive effects. (15 refs.)

Price, M. E. Why NICU nurses burn out and how to prevent it. *Contemporary OB/GYN,* 1979 (Mar.), *13,* 37-46. Reports on interviews with neonatologists and nursing administrators that indicate an alarming turnover rate among NICU nurses. Proposes that causes of burnout include lack of preparation to deal with bureaucracy and the extreme emotional strain of caring for critically ill infants. Suggests several solutions for burnout, including rotation to less emotionally stressful nursing duties, flexibility in work schedules, and opportunities for continuing education.

Readers report on the tragedy of burnout. *Learning,* April 1979, *7*(8), 76-77. Reports on a poll taken by the journal in January 1979. Of the 1,282 teachers who responded, 93 percent reported experiencing feelings related to burnout. Presents many anecdotes of burnout and of successful coping. Sixty-six percent of the teachers said they had discovered ways of coping, 24 percent were planning to quit the profession, and 7 percent said they were considering quitting.

Reed, S. What you can do to prevent teacher burnout. *National Elementary Principal,* 1979, *58,* 67-70. Outlines ways school principals can help prevent teacher burnout. Suggestions include: have teachers change to different grades, build self-esteem through positive reinforcement, involve teachers in decision making, communicate with each staff member, push for professional growth, promote physical and mental well-being, release the pressure, actively involve parents, and keep yourself tuned up.

Ricken, R. Teacher burnout: A failure of the supervisory process. *NASSP Bulletin,* 1980, *64*(434), 21-24. Discusses teacher burnout as stemming from both individual and system sources. Suggests that teachers get bogged down in the boring and tedious aspects of the job and that some become too secure so they do not try to keep their job fresh. Blames too rigid bureaucracy for stifling creativity of good teachers.

Ritter, C. When mothers burn out. *The Plain Truth,* 1977, *42*(4), 16-19; 35. Applies basic burnout concepts to the "nonprofessional" helping role of mother. Offers preventative measures and remedies that focus on more time for self, open communication, and more father-child involvement. (4 refs.)

Savicki, V., & Cooley, E. Theoretical and research considerations of burnout. *Children and Youth Services Review,* in press. Discusses problems in defining the concept of burnout and explores the implications of these definitions for training and treatment. Suggests directions for future research, with an emphasis on the role of individual characteristics in burnout and on the need for longitudinal studies. (37 refs.)

Scrivens, R. The big click. *Today's Education,* 1979, *68*(4), 34-35. Lists causes of teacher burnout, including: length of time on the job with the same routine, professional disillusionment, inadequate pay, inability to cope with changing educational methods, involvement with students' problems.

Seiderman, S. Combatting staff burnout. *Day Care and Early Education,* 1978, *5*(4), 6-9. Describes early symptoms of burnout among day-care workers. Suggestions for combatting burnout include: recognition of the problem, open communication system, staff involvement in operational problem solving, attention to working conditions, changes in routine and rhythm, combination of seriousness and fun, flexible job responsibilities, renewal experience, opportunities to experience success, responsible selfishness. (14 refs.)

Shannon, C., & Saleebey, D. Training child welfare workers to cope with burnout. *Child Welfare,* 1980, *59,* 463-468. Discusses workshop format designed to ease the experience of burnout. Forty-one child welfare workers and supervisors participated in a six-session workshop. According to participant evaluations, the most valuable aspects of workshop were learning to relax and receiving information about job stress and burnout. (8 refs.)

Shaw, S., Bensky, J. M., Dixon, B., & Bonneau, R. Strategies for dealing with burnout among special educators. *Education Unlimited,* 1980, *2*(4), 21-23. Proposes that the greatest source of stress is the discrepancy between teachers' expectations and others' expectations for the teacher role. Recommends several approaches to reducing burnout, including: (a) negotiation and specification of role and student load for special educators; (b) provision of complete job description for potential staff; (c) support services for staff; (d) job transfers; (e) positive feedback from administrators; (f) better management of special education policies and procedures. (13 refs.)

Shubin, S. Burnout: The professional hazard you face in nursing. *Nursing 78,* 1978, *8*(7), 22-27. Discusses basic concepts of burnout as they relate to nurses. Includes quotations about burnout symptoms and remedies from professionals in various fields.

Skinner, K. Burn-out: Is nursing dangerous to your health? *Journal of Nursing Care,* Dec. 1979, *12,* 8-30. Describes the burnout syndrome in terms of the nursing profession. Suggests several strategies for dealing with burnout, including self-analysis, work breaks, relaxation techniques, social support, physical exercise, changes in work routines, and getting a new job.

Smith, D., & McWilliams, L. Diagnostic-prescriptive approach to reading teacher burnout. *Reading World,* 1980, *20*(1), 53-56. Discusses factors considered to contribute to burnout among reading teachers: restrictive work routines, lack of opportunity for personal creativity, intangible and extremely time-consuming progress, budget cutbacks, public questioning of teacher competency. Gives nine suggestions for keeping work "fresh" and six suggestions for personal changes. (3 refs.)

Smits, S. J. Beyond "burnout." *Journal of Rehabilitation Administration,* February 1979, *3,* 2-3. Makes an editorial plea for greater attention to the causes of burnout so that actions can be taken to prevent it (rather than just treat it). Considers personal versus organizational causes in the area of rehabilitation, and questions whether there is an adequate "fit" between the nature of the work, the personnel, and existing organizations. (1 ref.)

Solomon, J. R. Additional perspectives on therapist burnout. *Social Casework,* 1979, *60*(3), 177-178. Offers additions to Larson, Gilbertson, and Powell

(1978). Argues that "career crisis" is an important but different phenomenon from burnout. Takes issue with previous view that isolation contributes to rapid burnout.

Sparks, D. Teacher burnout: A teacher center tackles the issue. *Today's Education,* 1979, *68*(4), 37-39. Discusses program developed by the Northwest Staff Development Center, which deals with teacher stress and burnout. Describes one of the Center's seven workshops (entitled "Stress and the Classroom Teacher") and gives an address for obtaining workshop materials.

Stewart, M. S., & Meszaros, P. S. What's your burnout score? *Journal of Home Economics,* 1981, *73*(3), 37-39. Gives brief description of burnout. Offers a checklist for assessing one's knowledge of the subject and one's degree of experienced burnout. Uses "burnout game" to give graphic illustration of conditions and behaviors that contribute to burnout. (3 refs.)

Storlie, F. J. Burnout: The elaboration of a concept. *American Journal of Nursing,* 1979, *19*(12), 2108-11. Discusses burnout as it relates to nursing and conceptualizes it as disillusionment. Offers anecdotes from nurses about incidents that cause disillusionment. Describes ten ideal job characteristics of nursing that could be deterrents to burnout. Discusses the intensive care unit nurse as being particularly vulnerable to burnout. (7 refs.)

Sullivan, R. C. The burn-out syndrome. *Journal of Autism and Developmental Disorders,* 1979, *9,* 112-117. Discusses causes of burnout in teachers and parents of autistic children, including: lack of respite, feelings of inability to effect significant change in the life of the child, lack of adequate coping skills, agency insensitivity. Ten pages of responses from parents and teachers follow the article. (8 refs.)

Teacher burnout: How to cope when your world goes black. *Instructor,* January 1979, pp. 56-62. Anecdotes from various teachers and other professionals in the field of education about the causes, prevention, and cure of burnout. Briefly defines mild, medium, and severe burnout. Looks at adult life cycles and their effects on teachers. Offers ten "commandments" to prevent teacher burnout. (5 refs.)

Thompson, J. W. "Burnout" in group home houseparents. *American Journal of Psychiatry,* 1980, *137*(6), 710-714. Reports results of survey study of forty-seven house parents of group homes for emotionally disturbed adolescents. For males, high burnout correlated with salary level, screening prospective residents, and having no decision-making power in accepting residents. For females, high burnout correlated with screening prospective residents and running group meetings with residents. For both sexes, low burnout correlated with support from friends and the board of directors of the group homes. (12 refs.)

Tiedeman, D. V. Burning and copping out of counseling. *Personnel and Guidance Journal,* 1979, *57,* 328-330. Offers criticism of Warnath and Shelton's (1976) view that situational factors, particularly inadequate education, are the major factors in burnout. Proposes that psychological problems are in both situations and individuals. Objects to earlier propositions that excuse individuals from appropriate implication in the dilemmas of their lives and careers. (3 refs.)

Valle, S. K. Burnout: Occupational hazard for counselors. *Alcohol Health and Research World,* 1979, *3,* 10-14. Discusses assumptions made by alcoholism counselors that contribute to burnout: (a) a counselor should be "together" at all times; (b) helping another alcoholic attain sobriety is fulfilling and is, of itself, sufficiently rewarding; (c) counselors' efforts will always be appreciated by clients; (d) being a recovered alcoholic automatically makes one a good counselor; (e) there is status and prestige in the job; (f) counselors can devote 100 percent of their time and efforts to working with clients. Suggests preventative measures.

Van Auken, S. Youth counselor burnout. *Personnel and Guidance Journal,* 1979, *58,* 143-144. Gives anecdotal evidence of youth counselor burnout. Suggests preventative measures, including: avoid being taken in by parents seeking to abdicate their responsibilities, keep meetings brief, maintain a sense of humor, consider the least dramatic steps first, and keep a clear picture of your professional objectives.

Veninga, R. Administrator burnout: Causes and cures. *Hospital Progress,* 1979, *60,* 45-52. Proposes that burnout among administrators arises from frustrating life "scripts" and/or organizational pressures. Scripts that can contribute to work frustration are: (a) trust only yourself; (b) everyone should see the world as I do; (c) I'm going to succeed even if it kills me. Discusses burnout symptoms and preventative measures.

Walsh, D. Classroom stress and teacher burnout. *Phi Delta Kappan,* 1979, *61*(4), 253. Gives brief review of symptoms and causes of burnout among teachers.

Warnath, C. F. Counselor burnout: Existential crisis or a problem for the profession? *Personnel and Guidance Journal,* 1979, *57,* 325-328. Responds to Tiedeman's (1979) view that Warnath and Shelton (1976) put too much emphasis on situational factors affecting burnout and not enough emphasis on individual responsibility. Reiterates that social context may contribute greatly to burnout and may also hold many of the resources for "curing" burnout. Contends that counselor education is not reality oriented enough and that counselor-educators must become more aware of the applicability of what they are teaching to the job settings in which their graduates work. (4 refs.)

Warnath, C. F., & Shelton, J. L. The ultimate disappointment: The burned out counselor. *Personnel and Guidance Journal,* 1976, *55,* 172-175. Discusses conditions leading to counselor burnout, including: (a) the split between philosophy and practice during the graduate school experience, (b) the lack of openness of teachers and counselors about their feelings related to burnout, (c) the gap between ideals and job realities, (d) little reinforcement from clients or colleagues, (e) bureaucratic demands. Gives eight suggestions for system changes. (3 refs.)

Weiskopf, P. E. Burnout among teachers of exceptional children. *Exceptional Children,* 1980, *47*(1), 18-24. Discusses environmental sources of stress that may contribute to burnout in teachers of exceptional children, including: work overload, lack of perceived success, amount of direct contact with children, staff-child ratio, program structure, responsibility for others. Gives nine suggestions for prevention. (15 refs.)

Wise, T. N., & Berlin, R. M. Burnout: Stresses in consultation-liaison psychiatry. *Psychosomatics,* 1981, *22,* 744-751. Discusses stresses of consultation-liaison psychiatry that foster burnout, including: (a) role ambiguity and conflict; (b) difficult patients; (c) devaluation of psychiatrist by other physicians; (d) poor working conditions. Suggests several prevention strategies, including: (a) peer-group support; (b) effective leadership by the consultation-liaison division head; (c) regular assessment of goals; (d) a flexible approach; (e) balance of consultation and liaison activities; (f) opportunities for ongoing research activities. (25 refs.)

Zabel, R. H., & Zabel, M. K. Burnout: A critical issue for educators. *Education Unlimited,* March 1980, *2,* 23-25. Describes burnout syndrome among special education teachers. Discusses techniques for reducing burnout, including reduction of student-teacher ratio, shorter work hours, opportunities for time out, shared student load, and training in stress management. (3 refs.)

Zahn, J. Burnout in adult educators. *Lifelong Learning: The Adult Years,* 1980, *4*(4), 4-6. Describes the general characteristics of burnout and discusses the following contributors to teacher burnout: lack of adequate preparation, monotony, and feelings of helplessness. Suggests several remedies for burnout. (5 refs.)

BOOKS AND MONOGRAPHS

Cherniss, C. *Professional burnout in human service organizations.* New York: Praeger, 1980.

Cherniss, C. *Staff burnout: Job stress in the human services.* Beverly Hills, Calif.: Sage Publications, 1980.

Edelwich, J., with Brodsky, A. *Burn-out: Stages of disillusionment in the helping professions.* New York: Human Sciences Press, 1980.

Freudenberger, H. J. *The staff burn-out syndrome.* Washington, D.C.: Drug Abuse Council, 1975.

Freudenberger, H. J., with Richelson, G. *Burn-out: The high cost of high achievement.* Garden City, N.Y.: Anchor Press, 1980.

Jones, J. W. (Ed.), *The burnout syndrome: Current research, theory, interventions.* Park Ridge, Ill.: London House Press, 1981.

Klein, M. J., & Atcom staff. *Burnout: What it is, how it affects you, what you can do to prevent it.* New York: Atcom, 1979.

Levine, G. *I quit!: A guide to burn out prevention.* Orange, Calif.: Indeco, 1981.

Maslach, C., & Jackson, S. E. *The Maslach Burnout Inventory.* Research ed. Palo Alto, Calif.: Consulting Psychologists Press, 1981.

Moracco, J. C. *Burnout in counselors and organizations.* Ann Arbor, Mich.: ERIC-CAPS, 1981.

Paine, W. (Ed.), *Job stress and burnout.* Beverly Hills, Calif.: Sage Publications, 1982.

Pines, A. M., & Aronson, E., with Kafry, D. *Burnout: From tedium to personal growth.* New York: Free Press, 1981.

Potter, B. A. *Beating job burnout.* San Francisco: Harbor/Putnam, 1980.

Reid, K. E. (Ed.), *Burnout in the helping professions.* Kalamazoo, Mich.: Western Michigan University, 1979.

Spaniol, L., & Caputo, J. *Professional burn-out: A personal survival kit.* Lexington, Mass.: Human Services Associates, 1979.

Truch, S. *Teacher burnout and what do about it.* Novato, Calif.: Academic Therapy Publications, 1980.

Vash, C. *The burnt-out administrator.* New York: Springer, 1980.

Veninga, R. L., & Spradley, J. P. *The work/stress connection: How to cope with job burnout.* Boston: Little, Brown, 1981.

White, W. L. *Incest in the organizational family: The unspoken issue in staff and program burn-out.* Rockville, Md.: HCS, Inc., 1978.

White, W. L. *A systems response to staff burn-out.* Rockville, Md.: HCS, Inc., 1978.

White, W. L. *Relapse as a phenomenon of staff burn-out among recovering substance abusers.* Rockville, Md.: HCS, Inc., 1979.

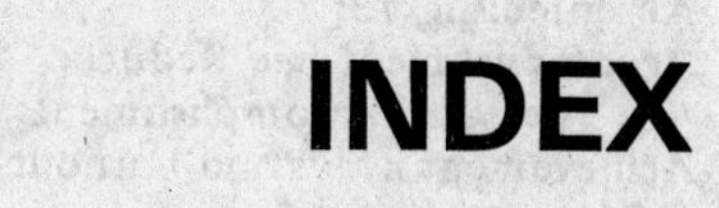

INDEX